NURS
QUAL...
MEASUREMENT

NURSING QUALITY MEASUREMENT

Quality Assurance Methods for Peer Review

Edited by
ALAN PEARSON

With contributions from
ANNE WILES, LEONARD A GOLDSTONE, SUE BRADSHAW,
PAUL WAINWRIGHT

An H M & M Nursing Publication

JOHN WILEY & SONS

Chichester · New York · Brisbane · Toronto · Singapore

© John Wiley & Sons Ltd 1987

H M & M Publishers is an imprint of John Wiley & Sons Ltd, Baffins Lane, Chichester, Sussex PO19 1UD, England.

British Library Cataloguing in Publication Data

Nursing quality measurement: quality
   assurance methods for peer review.
   1. Nursing—Quality control
   2. Quality assurance
   I. Pearson, Alan, 1948–   II. Wiles, Anne
   610.73′068′5   RT85.5

ISBN 0 471 91589 0

Library of Congress Cataloging in Publication Data

Nursing quality measurement.

   (An H M + M nursing publication)
   1. Nursing audit. 2. Nursing—Quality control.
3. Peer review. I. Pearson, Alan. II. Wiles, Anne.
III. Series: An HM+M nursing publication. [DNLM:
1. Nursing. 2. Quality Assurance, Health Care.
3. Peer Review. WY 16 N9787]
RT85.5.N8664   1987   362.1′73   87–8194
ISBN 0 471 91589 0 (pbk.)

Typeset by Woodfield Graphics, Arundel, West Sussex.
Printed and bound in Great Britain by Biddles Ltd, Guildford, Surrey

Table of Contents

Contributors

ALAN PEARSON PhD MSc SRN ONC RNT DipNEd DANS FRCN (Editor), Professor of Nursing, Deakin University, Geelong, Victoria, Australia; formerly Senior Nurse, Clinical Practice Development, Burford and Oxford Nursing Development Unit.

PAUL WAINWRIGHT MSc SRN RCNT RNT DANS, Assistant Director of Standards, Southend Health Authority.

ANNE WILES MSc SRN RCNT RNT DANS, Tutor, Oxford School of Nursing.

LEONARD GOLDSTONE BA (Econ) Hons MSc FSS, Head of School of Health Studies, Newcastle upon Tyne Polytechnic.

SUE BRADSHAW SRN, Senior Nurse, Geriatrics, Oxfordshire Health Authority.

Preface

'Quality Assurance' is rapidly becoming a part of the vocabulary of those who manage health services. As services become more and more expensive and sophisticated, and patients or clients become increasingly involved in their own health, it is right that attention should be focused on attempts to set acceptable standards of quality, and to create programmes to monitor quality.

There is a tendency in nursing, however, to charge nurse managers with the task of setting standards or monitoring them, and a recent trend is to involve non-nurses in monitoring the work of nurses. Whilst the organisation in which nurses work has a responsibility to ensure that adequate standards are maintained, the notion of quality assurance can be used in a creative way by clinical nurses. Unfortunately, many clinical nurses know little about setting standards and measuring quality, or, if they do know about it, see it as something which managers impose on them.

Setting standards and devising tools and programmes to measure quality is legitimately the role of nurses who are involved in the daily delivery of nursing care. This book aims at presenting the idea of setting standards, and exploring a number of methods of quality measurement. It is written specifically for clinical nurses, and argues that quality assurance in nursing must be seen as a form of peer review whereby experienced nurse clinicians use developed tools to review each other's work. When used in this way, measuring the quality of nursing can become much more than a form of control by organisations and their managements – it can become an effective method of generating change in clinical practice which will enable nursing to deliver the high standards which it has traditionally striven for, and thus have real benefits for those who receive the services of professional nurses.

All the contributors have both in-depth experience of attempting to measure quality and a genuine desire to help clinical nurses to monitor and improve their standards. Our hope is that clinical nurses themselves will become more interested and involved in developing quality assurance programmes, and that the current trend in setting up such programmes will end up with an improvement in the quality of care giving, rather than simply an improvement in measuring care. Quality *assurance* implies that the end result of such programmes will be the ability to promise the patient or client that an acceptable standard will be maintained. Without the active involvement of the direct care-giving nurse, the promise will be no more than one which will *measure* quality, with no guarantee that care will change.

ALAN PEARSON
1987

Acknowledgements

Every book is a combination of ideas held in the author's head which have been acquired from many experiences, and many other people. Those who have contributed to the development of these ideas will see themselves in this book, and although they are too numerous to name, the contribution of our mentors is acknowledged.

Thanks are due to the following for permission to include their original work in this overview of methods:

Appleton-Century-Crofts – *Nursing Audit*: QUALPACS

Loeb Centre for Nursing – *Patient Service Checklist*

Newcastle upon Tyne Polytchnic Products Limited, Library, Ellison Building, Ellison Place, Newcastle upon Tyne, NE1 8ST

Finally we acknowledge the input of the following: nurses and patients involved in applying these methods in practice; Liz Crabtree who painstakingly typed the manuscript, and Anne Wiles, Sue Bradshaw, Kate Wood, Sue Pembrey and Malcolm Ross for permission to reproduce the material on Oxfordshire's Quality Assurance programme.

AP

1
Nursing and Quality

ALAN PEARSON

About This Book

The purpose of this book is to give a broad overview of the practical use of tools to measure quality, and of ways in which clinical nurses can use them to raise quality. This first chapter is a general introduction and explanation of quality assurance, concepts related to quality assurance, and how quality assurance is inextricably linked to the work of clinical nurses. Chapter 2 explores the subject of peer review – that is, where professionals of equal standing attempt to look at each other's work in order to determine its quality. In the case of nursing, quality assurance tools can be used by clinical nurses to review and assess other's work as a group of peers. Chapters 3–6 consider four specific approaches to assessing quality. There are other approaches and tools currently being implemented in nursing throughout the world, and thus the book is not a comprehensive overview of quality assurance in nursing but aims at presenting approaches which are gaining popularity and are being used in practice. The final two chapters discuss introducing change, and present an example of the introduction of a quality assurance programme. It is hoped that the reader will be able to acquire a basic understanding of quality assurance, and an appreciation of the need to involve clinical nurses closely in implementing a programme.

Quality Assurance – an introduction

Every organisation has a responsibility to monitor the quality of its activities, to aim to maintain satisfactory standards and to raise them where appropriate. The health service, and nursing as a component of that service, is now under pressure to introduce methods to aim at 'assuring quality'. The terms 'quality assurance' and 'quality control' are increasingly becoming part of the current nursing vocabulary. 'Quality' is defined by the King's English Dictionary (1930) as 'nature or character of, in relation to right or wrong, as of an action; power of effects'. 'Assurance' is said to denote 'freedom from doubt' and 'control' is described as 'to regulate, to govern or direct'. Quality assurance may therefore be interpreted as promising, or making certain of, a standard of excellence. Control is the means by which quality can be assured. Mayers *et al* (1977) observe that quality assurance has the goal of making certain that nursing practices will produce good patient outcomes. The purpose of quality assurance is, according to Schmadl (1979), to assure the consumer of nursing of a specified degree of excellence through continuous measurement and evaluation.

Quality assurance has as its elements:

— measurement of quality (with standard setting inherent in this)
— evaluating care through judging measurements
— acting on the evaluation

Measurement is an objective process of ascertaining the dimensions, capacity or quantity of something, whilst evaluation is a subjective process which describes a judgement based on measurement (Schmadl 1979). Measuring and evaluating are not the sole components of quality assurance. They are a means of instituting change in order to improve care – to raise *standards* or increase quality

Measuring and evaluating

In order to measure and evaluate, or make a judgement, about such a complex activity as nursing, it is important to see the task in some organised way. In simple terms, quality assurance involves deciding what *should* be, comparing what *should* be with reality, and identifying the gaps and taking action. Whilst the third step involves a degree of subjective judgement, it is comparatively simple if the first two steps are completed. The first two steps, however, are extremely difficult to complete.

To measure what *should* be involves identifying *standards* and *criteria*. A standard has been defined as 'a measure to which others conform' (Crow 1981) or 'the desired levels of achievement' (Schroeder & Maibusch 1984). A standard is therefore the level which others accept as the baseline for good practice. A criterion has been defined as 'a statement which is measurable, reflecting the intent of a standard' (Lang 1979). Continence, pain, personal hygiene are all examples of criteria appropriate to nursing patients. Using the criterion of personal hygiene, a standard which may be agreed on may be 'the patient is clean and says she feels comfortable'. Thus, before being able to measure and evaluate, a decision on what needs to be measured is needed (ie. criteria have to be agreed upon). Once the criteria have been identified, standards then must be set. The standard becomes what *should* be; and measurement then enables an assessor to establish whether or not the reality of care meets that standard.

Criteria

Jelinek, Haussman & Hegyvary (1974) identify the three broad criteria which can be approached to measure quality:

— structural approach
— process approach
— outcome approach

Structure

The structural approach focuses upon the prerequisites for patient care, which include the physical facilities, the organisation of the unit or institution and the resources, both human and other. Any investigation of these areas should indicate the predispositions for, and the constraints against, high quality care.

Process

The process approach applies itself to the actual carrying out of care, and focuses on the nurse, her intellectual processes and her behaviour as it relates directly to the patient and to other members of staff. Measurement is of those activities that are related to the quality of nursing care for which they are accountable.

Outcome

The outcome approach looks at the patient's behaviour, health status, knowledge, or other predetermined factor, when his/her nursing is completed, with the intention of seeing if the effect of nursing care has been successful. The approach concentrates on the patient's welfare and the ultimate outcome of care, including recovery and mortality rates and some estimations of patient satisfaction.

Basically, these three approaches cannot be separated, because in order to assess quality effectively, information about –

the resources available (STRUCTURE)
how they are used (PROCESS)
and the eventual effects (OUTCOME)

needs to be collected before a judgement of quality can be made. Structure, process and outcome are therefore three parts of a whole, and cannot be divorced from each other in reality (Fig. 1.1)

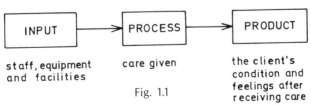

Fig. 1.1

Setting standards

Standards are the 'point of reference' which underpin any exercise in quality assurance in the same way that the speedometer in a car underpins the drivers capacity to know what speed she is travelling at.

An attempt to set standards relating to an apparently simple task such as the giving of medication may read something like this:

MAXIMUM: All patients will take own medicines at the correct time and dosage, witnessed by a nurse, and will be able to explain the nature of the medication when asked, except when there is evidence that they are physically or intellectually unable to do so.   EXCELLENCE (extremely good)

OPTIMUM: All patients will be given the correct medication at the correct time and be able to explain the nature of the medication when asked, except when there is evidence that they are physically or intellectually unable to do so.   DESIRABLE (good)

MINIMUM: All patients will be given the correct medication at the correct time.   ACCEPTABLE (OK)

NOT ACCEPTABLE (bad)

Because standards relate to magnitude, they assume unacceptable practice and highest possible practice. Although the Royal College of Nursing documents refer to 'acceptable levels of excellence' (RCN 1980; 1981) and other writers use this idea, excellence can be seen as the highest possible practice. So, a standard can be seen to be a level of performance or provision which is unacceptable, acceptable, the optimum, or excellent and is related to criteria which are regarded as being legitimate areas for determining overall success.

The division of standards into the three discrete areas of structure, process and outcome has been used by many nurses in their pursuit of setting acceptable standards. Clarke (1984) asserts that, given these three areas, and specific criteria, standard statements can be made which are 'observable, measurable and reasonable'. She gives the following examples of standard statements, using this framework:

The client's access to the health visitor:

	Structure	Process	Outcome
MAXIMUM LEVEL (excellence)	Health visitor carries a bleep on which she can be contacted at any time when a patient or relative phones	Health visitor explains her function, pattern of work, and the means of contacting her to every client at the time of first contact and informs the client of any changes	Any client who requests a visit will be visited on the same day that the request is made
MINIMUM LEVEL (acceptable)	Health visitor has a telephone at which someone is available to answer calls between 9 and 10 in the morning every day from Monday to Friday	Health visitor gives a telephone number to each new client at the first contact	Any client will be able to speak to a health visitor (not necessarily his own) within 24 hours of the original request

Standard-setting is extremely difficult and needs to be dynamic because changes in knowledge also mean changes in acceptable standards. And the subjective nature of nursing someone is surrounded by the immeasurable areas of values, attitudes and opinion, which make up professional judgement. Trying to write down standard statements not only takes a great deal of time, but the selection of acceptable criteria is difficult because there are huge differences between what nurses think nursing is, who needs nursing, when nursing is needed and who should nurse. Furthermore, one nurse's acceptable standard is another's view of Utopian excellence, which may be seen as an unacceptable standard by yet another.

The example of giving medication used earlier would no doubt be the subject of much discussion and criticism in a group of nurses. Is it, for example, acceptable that only the medication should be given, regardless of whether the patient understands what is happening or not? Is it excellent that patients take their own drugs or is the possibility of loss of control inherent in such an approach an indicator of unacceptability? Then there is the problem of generalising about the individuals who nurses nurse, and the ethical issues involved in judging whether the patient suffering from a terminal illness is able to 'take' the news, or if he is 'emotionally' unable to take it, and therefore has not been told what this drug is meant to do. And who should be involved in setting standards? Should it be nurses, should it be consumers, should it be both? Some studies suggest that members of the public would probably set very low standards for nursing; their expectations are low and they are based on previous experience of nursing. In evaluating nursing care, the majority of consumers have nothing to compare it with. For example, patients interviewed in one study (Pearson 1985) regarded the depersonalising leading from rigid task assignment and routinisation as entirely acceptable, and valued it highly because it was perceived as being efficient and symbolic of good nursing.

In discussing the involvement of patients in evaluating nursing, Hall (1966) asks 'Can we do this by examining the product, ie. the patient on discharge? Too often we know that the patient recovers in spite of the care he experiences. Can we find out the quality by asking the patient his opinion of it? He may be able to tell us his reactions to the kind he has experienced but unless he has experienced and understood each kind, he will be in no position to help us evaluate'. If it is only nurses, which nurses – managers, practitioners, educators? Hall (1966) argues that setting minimum standards must be the province of committed, educated nurses, who are primarily involved in nursing patients, but who draw on the consumer groups, and on the expertise of managers, researchers and teachers.

Although the task is onerous, groups of nurses, predominantly clinical, but including managers and educators, are the logical source of standard statements, provided that they actively seek validation of their ideas with members of the public and from other workers who make up the multidisciplinary team.

The RCN (1980) says:

> 'Statements related to nursing care can only be valid if set by those familar with the values, objectives and practice of nursing care and it is the responsibility of the nursing profession alone to agree an acceptable level of excellence'.

The second report from this committee (RCN 1981) acknowledged the difficulty in developing standards which could be used by the profession as a whole to consider and agree on acceptable levels of excellence. The committee's aim was to look at the values seen to be essential to nursing and then to translate these values into explicit standard statements. They emphasised the importance of the use of a systematic approach to care and presented three areas for consideration:

(a)   the nursing care of each patient should be individually planned, the plan being based on an assessment of individual needs.
(b)   the care given should be systematically recorded and subsequently reviewed to see how far the goals have been reached.
(c)   the individual nurse should accept accountability for her individual nursing action.

No criteria by which to judge the level of achievement of such standards were offered, however. The committee suggested that norms, check lists, and so on were inadequate and inappropriate. Whilst the formulation of clear standard statements from a united nursing profession would be a wonderful development, it would seem that this is impossible. What perhaps is possible, is to continue the committee's translation of current values into explicit standard statements and to encourage nurses to use them as a basis for evaluating patient care.

Whilst the nursing process and individual accountability of the clinical nurse are becoming highly valued in the current ideology of nursing, there are many other issues such as the right of the patient to informed choice, to participation in care planning and to preserve his own life style. Such values can be translated into broad standards and this is the first step for nurses to take when beginning to set criteria to measure levels of achievement.

More importantly, however, the second report from the RCN (1981) sees setting standards as an everyday part of nurses' work. Maybe it is at this level that the real setting of acceptable standards and standards of excellence can be developed. But widespread, locally set-up standards and quality assurance efforts involving those who nurse are the crucial element in developing standards which will actually influence practice. The meaning of standards must be clear to those who they are created to help and who must agree with them.

Broad universal standards are essential, but specific, operational standards have the inherent possibility of really raising the level of care which finally reaches the patient.

Standards of excellence are important, because without them nurses would lose direction, but for the time being, achieving excellence may still be Utopian. The current state of nursing may demand that nurses can only reach minimally acceptable standards. Pembrey (1984) says that an acceptable standard can only be achieved if the giver of care is competent enough to do so. She says:

> 'Standards of competent nursing are not reached reliably by untrained people or those who are in training. Furthermore, maintaining professional standards of competence requires frequent practice and continuing mastery of new knowledge and skills. The standard of professional work depends on two things: qualified practitioners and the quality of the professional education in both the initial preparation and the continuing mastery of the discipline throughout professional life'.

Standards, criterion and quality assurance

Quality assurance is an attempt to promise quality to the receivers of nursing. It relates directly to the identification of criterion and standards, and the construction of tools to assess whether or not standards are achieved. Finally, it leads to action which will promote the achievement of agreed standards. Figure 1.2 (overleaf) outlines how this process can be visualised.

Current approaches to quality assurance

There is a growing literature on quality assurance, and a number of tools have been developed and are in use: the most popular of these are discussed in detail in following chapters. All approaches are based on criteria and standards established by their authors, and all can be categorised into the structure/process/outcome framework. There is still much debate on how tools should be constructed, and on the virtues of choosing, for example, to focus on process or outcome.

Hall (1966) points out that 'prior to any discussion of the quality of nursing care, one must determine what it is that is being evaluated "What is nursing?"'. She goes on to ask 'What methods can we use to evaluate the quality of nursing

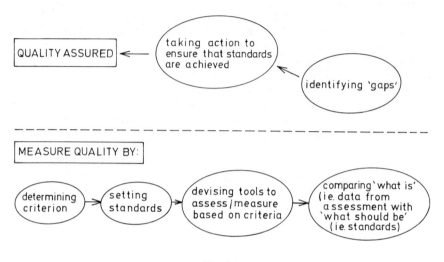

Fig. 1.2

care? Can we do this by examining the product, i.e. the patient on discharge? Can we find out the quality by asking the patient his opinion of it? He may be able to tell us his reactions to the kind he has experienced but unless he has experienced and understood each kind, he will be in no position to help us evaluate. It seems that the most valid method lies in the observation of the process itself'. Hegyvary & Haussman (1976) concur with this view, proposing that the most valid measurement of the quality of nursing is that which focuses on the actual nursing performed in the delivery of care to a patient. The above statement by Hall, however, lays the field open for extensive discussion on how best to measure quality, a topic which is widely discussed and argued about in all fields of nursing.

Bloch (1975), Mayers et al (1977), and Doughty & Mash (1977) all suggest a combination of the process-evaluation and outcome-evaluation approaches to constitute a process-outcome approach. This combination may describe the extent to which the achievement of objectives is due to the nursing given.

Much has been written on the 'best' method of quality care evaluation, and various writers argue in favour of a specific approach whilst validly criticising methods which do not meet their approval. It is reasonable to suggest that an effective quality assurance programme may need to use several methods, and that, indeed, to do so may increase effectiveness (Hover & Zimmer 1978). Methods encompassing a structure, process, and outcome approach may be those of choice for nursing, exploring, as they do, the activity within the unit and its effect on the ultimate outcomes.

The use of such a combination will allow the nursing process, and outcomes, to be evaluated, both concurrently and retrospectively, in the drive with which nurses have traditionally identified – to improve and maintain the quality of care they provide (Egleston, 1980).

Quality assurance tools

Tools used in quality assurance are essentially data collection instruments. Two methods of data collection are identified in the literature – retrospective and concurrent. The former utilises a review of the nursing given after it is completed, whereas the latter takes place whilst the nursing is still in progress. Retrospective evaluation of the quality of nursing may be effected (Mayers et al 1977) by:

— post-care patient interview
— post-care patient questionnaire
— post-care staff conference
— audit of the records.

Concurrent evaluation may be effected by:

— assessment of the outcomes of care
— patient interview
— conference between patient, staff and relatives
— direct observation of care
— measurement of the competency of the nurse
— audit of the records

Methods of retrospective evaluation

Post-care patient interview/questionnaire The patient interview and question-naire involve the evaluator in obtaining information from the patient and his family, on or after discharge. These methods are designed to measure the level of patient satisfaction, but have disadvantages in that the patient may remember recent events clearly, forgetting those which occurred during a previous and perhaps more intensive period of care.

Some outcomes of care may also be determined by the use of judicious questioning, as well as from the patient's satisfaction. Raphael's (1967) inter-views of staff and patients showed that patients' complaints were mainly concerned with lack of privacy and boredom, whereas the staff felt that the physical environment and equipment were unsatisfactory.

Post-care conference Post-care conferences should involve all members of the care team in critically analysing all aspects of a patient's care, including his response, progress and outcomes. This has the disadvantage that it may be less objective than an evaluation carried out by an uninvolved auditor.

Retrospective audit of the records The chart or record review appears, from the literature, to be the method most commonly employed and involves the systematic inspection of an agreed percentage of the records of patients dis-charged from care during a given length of time. The American Hospitals Association considers a review of all records to be necessary, but the J C A H recommends review of 'an adequate sample' (Zimmer 1974) without specifying what this may be.

Doughty & Mash (1977) believe that between one-third and a quarter of the annual discharge rate for a diagnosis always gives a representative sample. They also believe that an audit of the top 10–20 most commonly found dismissal diagnoses has an effect on a great deal of patient care. If smaller populations are to be investigated, Mayers *et al* (1977) say that '...the smaller the universe, the higher the percentage of charts needed to form a representative sample'. They also say that an audit which relies on chart review depends heavily upon good documentation of care. It is assumed that what is done is documented, and that what is documented has been performed or effected. Phaneuf (1976) claims that the conditions which lead to good documentation also lead to good nursing care, but Jelinek *et al* (1974) believe that nurses soon learn to make records which produce favourable results from an audit.

Methods of concurrent evaluation

Assessment of the outcomes of care   The assessment of care outcomes requires that the patient's present state be compared with a set of objectives. This concept is utilised by Mayers (1978) in her method for recording the patient's care plan and progress. It has also been used by Hilger (1974), who formulated a set of desired outcomes for the patient with a colostomy, and Anderson (1974), who defined categories of outcomes for patients suffering varying degrees of limitation due to congestive cardiac failure.

Patient interviews   Individual patients can be interviewed, or asked to complete a questionnaire whilst still receiving care. On the whole, this method is unpopular and is rarely used because patients tend to find it difficult to be honest in evaluating nursing whilst still receiving it.

Conference between patient, staff and relatives   Again, this is not widely used in quality assurance programmes, although it is used in care planning.

Direct observation of care   The observation of nursing care may centre upon the nurse and her behaviour or it may, as in the quality patient care scale of Wandelt & Ager (1974), involve the observation and rating of the care given to an individual patient, perhaps by a number of personnel. The latter method is used to assess the care given within a unit or a hospital, rather than that performed by an individual.

Measurement of the competency of the nurse   An assessment of the competency of an individual may involve the use of a performance instrument such as that of Tate, who measured the traits of a staff nurse, or those of Slater or Dyer, who formulated scales of nurse competency. (Jelinek, Haussman & Hegyvary 1974). Mayers *et al* (1977) believe that the personal traits of a carer are indirectly related to nursing care, but Hegyvary & Haussman (1976) ask whether a measure of the behaviour of a nurse, her creativity, tolerance or cheefulness, is a valid measure of nursing care quality or merely a measure of the personal characteristics of caregivers.

Audit of records   Audit of records involves the inspection of nursing records which are still in use, the assumption being made that the records accurately reflect the care given. Criticism has been made by Haussman & Hegyvary (1976) that this method simply improves documentation, not nursing care.

Much has been written on the 'best' method of quality care evaluation, various writers argue in favour of a specific approach whilst validly criticising methods which do not meet with their approval. It is reasonable to suggest that an effective quality assurance programme may need to use several methods and that, indeed, to do so may increase effectiveness (Hover & Zimmer 1978). Methods encompassing a structure, process, and outcome approach may be those of choice for nursing, exploring, as they do, the activity within nursing and its effect on the ultimate outcomes.

Determining the degree of quality of nursing desired, and ensuring that it is achieved, is an important part of the work of the clinical nurse, and appraisal of quality is a means of instituting necessary change in nursing practice. The whole process must be a continuous one of implementation of change and re-evaluation.

Setting standards, quality measurement, quality control, and quality assurance are thus different foci of measuring quality, and using this measurement to arrive at judgement of quality related to agreed standards. To promise the patient a good service, these must be accompanied by a process of change, where poor quality or low standards are raised.

Quality Assurance and the clinical nurse

'Clinical' nurses are those whose major role is to give a direct, professional service to patients or clients. They are people at the 'sharp end' of the health care system – the hands-on nurses who are the worker bees of the system. Since the beginning of modern nursing, these people have been part of a huge organisational hierarchy, and have been subordinate to nurse managers, doctors and administrators, yet it is they who deliver nursing, and hence it is they who will really determine how good or how bad nursing will be. The education they receive, and the organisational climate and resources available in the area in which they work does, of course, have a crucial impact on the standard of work. Thus, the quality of nursing is influenced by nurse educators, nurse managers, doctors and health service administrators, but even if all of these are of the highest order, the care itself is still determined by those who give it.

Furthermore, the 'experts' in giving nursing care are those who have chosen to make a career out of clincial practice, because expertise in clinical nursing is highly dependent upon actually doing it. Nursing in the western world, like many other practice disciplines, suffers from the overwhelming trend of devaluing practitioners and the tendency is for status to increase in proportion to the distance between the nurse and patient care: in other words, the further away from the patient, the greater the status and financial reward.

There is now a desire to arrest this trend, and practice developments in recent years have all focused on increasing the accountability of clinical nurses to the receiver of nursing, rather than to a hierarchy of superiors. In the final analysis, both professionally and in law, the clinical nurse is accountable for the care she prescribes and gives. The nurse is therefore bound, because of her position, to provide a standard of nursing care which is acceptable to society, to other members of her profession, and the health care system in general. In other words, the clinical nurse is really accountable for the quality of care she provides.

Health care is getting more complex every day, and the understanding and expectations of the patient – the customer or consumer – are increasing in complexity. It follows, then, that attempts by clincial nurses to maintain a satisfactory standard must also become much clearer, more comprehensive, and more visible. It is no longer sufficient for sister to claim that 'The standards on my ward are as high as anywhere else'. What is meant by standard? How can 'anywhere else' be compared with the ward in question? It is no longer acceptable to say that 'The quality of nursing care here is excellent'! What indicates that the nursing is of a high quality?

Nursing has an objective side to it – parts of its practice can be precisely measured and assessed, but much of nursing is subjective and difficult to measure. Knowing this, nurses are prone to dismiss ways of trying to set standards and measure quality: they hope that by emphasising the emotional investment between the nurse and patient, the drive to be more specific will go away. It is unlikely that this will ever happen: indeed, the pressure on nursing to be more accurate in assuring quality is likely to increase. If clinical nurses fail to grasp this, and continue to pay little attention to regulating their own practice, there are worrying indications that others will do it for them. If they really do want to be accountable for their practice, a greater interest and involvement in setting standards and assuring quality has become an urgent need.

Standard setting, quality measurement, evaluation of nursing and changing practice are the components of quality assurance. At the moment, few clinical nurses are interested or involved in developing quality assurance programmes, and this gives rise to the risk that they will be imposed on practitioners by administrators and nurse managers. Clinical nurses are, however, accountable for the care they provide, and are the best equipped to understand what needs to be measured, what criteria should be used, and to determine realistic standards. The essential element in quality assurance is ensuring that poor practice changes, and only clinical nurses can make this happen. This book therefore argues that quality assurance is a responsibility of clinical nurses, and should be seen as a tool for peer review.

In many organisations, quality is measured by nurse managers or other non-clinically involved nurses, using specific tools. If clinical nurses evaluated their colleagues:

— the results would carry more credibility
— the evaluators would gain insight into the shortcomings of their own practice
— the results would provide a basis for peer review
— and changes required to improve quality would therefore be more likely to occur

It is therefore essential that quality assurance should become a matter of concern for clinical nurses, and a part of day-to-day conversation in practice areas.

Using this book

This chapter has aimed at giving a broad overview of the issues and ideas involved in quality assurance, and to point out the central role of the clinical nurse in quality assurance. The rest of the book serves to present some tools which can be used as a basis for the setting up of a peer review system, discussed in Chapter 2. Some readers may find tools in the book that will help them, others may be led to discover different tools from the literature; whilst others may set out to identify criteria, set standards, and construct tools in their own workplace. It is hoped, however, that clinical nurses as a whole will be prompted to become much more involved with their managers and educators in the current drive to set standards and implement quality assurance in nursing.

References

Anderson M (1974) Development of outcome criteria for the patient with congestive heart failure. *Nursing Clinics of North America*, **9**(2)

Berg H (1974) Nursing audit and outcome criteria. *Nursing Clinics of North America*, **9**(2)

Bloch D (1975) Evaluation of nursing care in terms of process and outcome. *Nursing Research*, **24**(4)

Clark J (1984) Community nursing. *Lampada*, **1**, 13

Crow R (1981) Research and standards of nursing care: What is the relationship? *Journal of Advanced Nursing*, **6**, 491–496

Doughty D B & Mash N J (1977) *Nursing Audit*. Philadelphia: Davis

Egleston E M (1980) New J C A H standard on quality assurance *Nursing Research*, **29**(2), 113–114

Hall L E (1966) Another view of nursing care and quality. In Straub M & Parker K eds, *Continuity of Patient Care: the Role of Nurses*, 47–61. Washington D.C: Catholic University of America Press

Hegyvary S T & Haussman R K D (1976) Monitoring nursing care quality. *Journal of Nursing Administration*, **6**(9), 6–9

Hilger E (1974) Developing nursing outcome criteria *Nursing Clinics of North America*, **9**(2)

Hover J & Zimmer M J (1978) Nursing Quality assurance; the Wisconsin system. *Nursing Outlook*, **26**(4), 242–248

Jelinek D Haussman R & Hegyvary S (1974) *A Methodology for Monitoring Quality of Nursing Care*. Bethesda. U S Department of Health, Education and Welfare

King's English Dictionary (1930) London: British Book Company

Lang N (1976) Issues in Quality Assurance in Nursing. In *ANA Issues in Evaluative Research*. American Nurses Association

Longman Modern English Dictionary (1978) London: Longman

Mayers M (1978) *A Systematic Approach to the Nursing Care Plan*. New York: Appleton-Century-Crofts

Mayers M, Norby R B & Watson A B (1977) *Quality Assurance for Patient Care-Nursing Perspectives*. New York: Appleton-Century-Crofts

Pearson A (1985) *The Effects of Introducing New Norms in a Nursing Unit and an Analysis of the Process of Change.* Unpublished Ph D thesis, University of London: Goldsmiths' College, Department of Social Science and Administration

Pembrey S (1984) In praise of competence. *Lampada,* **2,** 12

Phaneuf M (1976) *The Nursing Audit.* New York: Appleton-Century-Crofts

Raphael W (1967) Do we know what patients think? *International Journal of Nursing Studies,* **4,** 209–223

Royal College of Nursing (1980) *Standards of Nursing Care.* London: R C N

Royal College of Nursing (1981) *Towards Standards.* London: R C N

Rowden R (1984) Quality Assurance. *Lampada,* **2,** 13

Schmadl J C (1979) Quality assurance: examination of the concept. *Nursing Outlook,* **27**(7), 462–465

Schroeder P S & Maisbusch R M (1984) *Nursing Quality Assurance – a Unit-based Approach.* Rockville: Aspen Systems Corporation

Wandelt M & Ager J (1974) *Quality Patient Care Scale.* New York: Appleton-Century-Crofts

Zimmer M J (1974) Quality assurance for outcomes of patient care. *Nursing Clinics of North America,* **9**(2)

2
Peer Review

PAUL WAINWRIGHT

One of the key issues in any quality assurance system is the question of who is going to set the standards and evaluate the quality. The medical profession are in no doubt as to who should review the quality of a doctor's work. In a monograph published by the Australian Hospital Association (1978) it is held that

> 'the patient is not equipped to judge the professional aspects of medical care, nor the competence of health professionals'

and

> 'it is not right for (health authorities and Government) to interfere in the professional aspects of medical care.
> ..... we are left with only one alternative if we believe some check should be made on the standards of care provided by doctors ..... this alternative is Peer Review – judgement and review by equals'.

The tone will be familiar to the British reader, and is well illustrated by references, in the courts and the reports of the Ombudsman, to 'clinical judgement', and in the operation of the General Medical Council and in systems such as the 'Three Wise Men'. In the United States, of course, there is a legal obligation on health care professions to 'institute measures' to ensure quality patient care (O'Loughlin & Kaulbach 1981) and this law 'mandates peer review for physicians'.

Cynics might argue that doctors not only reserve the right to be the sole judges of their own practice, but also feel quite able to control the content, and comment upon the quality of, the work of all other members of the health care team, and that nurses have aided and abetted this behaviour. However, there are

15

increasingly, in this country and abroad, attempts to argue that nursing has a unique, independent component and that the only people competent to evaluate the performance of a practising nurse are other practising nurses, her peers.

Definitions

The first problem is to define who exactly is a 'peer'. The Shorter Oxford English Dictionary defines a peer as

> 'an equal in standing or rank; one's equal before the law; an equal in any respect; one matched with another; a companion, mate; a rival'.

This is a pretty broad definition, but it clearly establishes the concept of equality. Furthermore, it allows that peers need not be equal in every respect. Phrases such as 'one's equal before the law; an equal in any respect' remind one of concepts such as the judicial 'jury of his peers' or the use of the term to denote those of the same age or the same year in school or university, while the sociologists talk of 'peer group pressure'.

For Beyers & Philips (1979), peer review involves 'registered nurses with the same role expectations or job descriptions or both', while Ramphal (1974) talks only of 'the evaluation by practising professional nurses of the quality of nursing care performed by other nurses according to stated norms of the profession'.

O'Loughlin & Kaulbach (1981) write that

> 'peer review can be defined as a process by which practitioners of the same rank, profession or setting critically appraise each other's work performance against established standards'

while to Lamberton et al (1977), peer review is

> 'an encounter between two individuals equal to one another in education, abilities, and qualifications, in which one person critically reviews the practice that the other has documented in a client's record'.

Mullins et al (1979) define peer review as

> 'the process used to appraise the quality of a registered nurse's professional performance and is conducted by a group of registered nurses who are actively engaged in some component of nursing practice'.

In the system described by Mullins et al a consumer representative also takes part in the process to reflect the nurses accountability to the client.

Finally, Maas & Jacox (1977) define the peer group as being all the registered nurses practising in the institution and describe peer review as

> 'the evaluation by practising professional nurses of the quality of services performed by other nurses, according to the standards established by the group'.

Purpose of peer review

It is clear from the previous section that, while there is basic agreement about what is meant by peer review, there are differences of interpretation. It might therefore be useful at this point to consider the uses to which peer review can be put.

Peer review is, quite clearly, about quality assurance. It also serves as the means by which the professional can go some way to discharging his accountability to his colleagues and his clients. It implies a willingness to open practice to scrutiny, to give an account of decisions and actions, and if necessary to justify and defend them. Such a view is supported by Passos (1973) who sees peer review as the hallmark of professionalism and the mechanism by which the nursing profession would be held accountable to society. Similar concepts are developed by Ciske *et al* (1983) who point out that peer review requires professional attitudes and behaviours towards peers, and by Maas & Jacox, who agree that peer review is necessary for demonstrating accountability for practice and who see it as an essential element of professional autonomy.

At its simplest level, peer review may be used informally by staff groups who meet together to discuss the way care is organised and delivered in their area, or who call upon colleagues in other areas for advice and consultancy. Examples might include the ward team who discuss together the relative merits of task allocation, patient allocation and primary nursing as means of organising care delivery, or who seek advice from colleagues in the psychogeriatric area on how best to manage a confused or demented surgical patient; or the young charge nurse who meets other ward managers at coffee and seeks their opinion on questions of ward organisation. Maas & Jacox, particularly, describe the informal development of such systems and their transition into more formal arrangements.

Peer review can, of course, be applied either to an individual or to a group or team. While both approaches form elements of quality control, the group approach can quite clearly be seen to be part of quality assurance, while the individual approach may be seen more as a management process, forming part of the appraisal system. Mullins *et al* (1979) list the purposes of peer review as follows:

1   To establish an objective means for providing evaluation feedback to individual nurses.
2   To recognise the individual nurse who has outstanding nursing skills and performs at a high level of clinical practice.
3   To identify individual areas of the nurse's practice needing further development.
4   To analyse the consistency of the individual nurse's practice compared to accepted professional standards.

while Beyers & Phillips (1979) say that the purpose of peer review is

'to measure the quality of care being given patients, to build on the strengths of the nurse being reviewed, and to identify the nurse's deficiencies or limitations to assist them in improving the quality of patient care given'.

They go on to say that 'the results of peer review may be used in determining advancements and salary increases'. Cleland (1983) is more specific about the use of peer review in areas such as salary awards:

'Under a system of peer review the collective recommendations might be, for example, that the top 30 per cent receive a merit increase, the middle 30 per cent a general increase, the lowest 30 per cent a warning, and finally, the lowest 10 per cent might not be recommended for contract renewal',

and Maas & Jacox describe the case of a nurse who was dismissed on the recommendation of a peer review committee.

Such an approach to peer review, while it is the logical conclusion of arguments that link peer review to professionalism and autonomy, would be difficult to develop within the present British health care system. However, recent political developments have made it less far-fetched an idea than it would have been even five years ago and we would be advised at least to have begun to consider the implications, prerequisites and consequences of such developments.

One difficulty associated with peer review of the individual nurse's provision of care to patients is that the organisation and delivery of care in many clinical settings is still fragmented and lacking in continuity, as well as being institutionalised and impersonal. It is therefore difficult to judge the work of an individual nurse on anything other than the technical skill with which she performs her work and the quality of the social interactions she has with patients, rather than on her skills of assessment, diagnosis and evaluation, or the extent to which she involves the patient in his care. In too many areas nursing is still a matter of 'doing what Sister tells you when she is there, and doing what you know she would do, when she is not there'.

A more fruitful approach, and one which might form an essential developmental step for the staff involved, would be to apply peer review to the functioning of a team of nurses, the staff of a ward or department. In view of the heterogeneous nature of the ward team in most British hospitals this approach stretches the definition of the peer group to the maximum, but it has the advantage of recognising the reality of our situation. Peer review of collective practice, rather than individual practice, can be confined to a particular aspect of care, as a form of problem-solving, or it might take an overall measure of quality such as Qualpacs or Phaneuf's Audit. The review can be carried out by the members of the team or by external reviewers who were selected by the team and identified as peers, and the findings of the review, fed back to the team members, would form the basis for future action such as education and training or changes in organisation and practice.

It is worth pointing out that peer review is also of great potential in nurse education. Used as part of the process of student assessment it provides students with the opportunity and the challenge of developing their critical faculties and their conceptual framework for quality and prepares them for the professional accountability required of them when qualified.

Who should perform peer review

We have already discussed definitions of 'peer' and 'the peer group' and noted that there are differences of opinion among various writers. Having considered the purpose of peer review, this is perhaps a good point to return to the question of who actually carries out the review.

The first consideration must be the acceptance of the reviewers by those reviewed. This would seem to be self-evident, but it is important to stress that if it is to succeed, a system of peer review cannot be imposed by a third party. The recognition of the need for peer review and the decision to develop a system must come from within the group and the responsibility for carrying out the review must rest within the group.

However, if we take literally some of the authors already cited, we are faced with the prospect of a very limited system. Beyers & Phillips, for example, refer to nurses 'with the same role expectation or job description or both'. They suggest, as an example, that theatre nurses should review the practice of theatre nurses, but their words could also be taken to mean that staff nurse should review staff nurse and enrolled nurse should review enrolled nurse. Similarly, O'Loughin & Kaulbach refer to 'practitioners of the same rank, profession, or setting' and Allbritten *et al* (1982) to 'individuals equal to one another in education, abilities, and qualifications'. Such constraints pose several problems.

For one thing, given the mixed and varied nature of British nursing, it might prove very difficult to provide sufficient peers by these criteria to make the system workable. For another, surely there is much to be gained from exposing one's practice to review by a colleague better qualified and more experienced than oneself? And finally there is the risk of tunnel vision and isolation if only a theatre nurse may review another theatre nurse, only a paediatric nurse may criticise other paediatric nurses.

Allbritten *et al* suggest that peer review is a one-to-one situation, but this would seem to be fraught with difficulties and dangers. On the other hand, Mullins *et al* describe a system in which the peer review committee consists of three clinical nurses of different degrees of experience, a nursing administrator, a member of the staff of the school of nursing, and a consumer. If peer review was established in an organisation to the extent that a peer review committee or committees existed this would seem a good model. The clinical nurse members could be co-opted from appropriate clinical settings to ensure that specialist practice could be reviewed objectively, while the administrator and teacher would presumably bring the benefits of seniority, experience and higher education.

To return to the subject of collective practice, a lot will depend on the nature of any tools or standards to be used. For example, if Qualpacs is chosen by the staff as an acceptable measure of quality, there would probably be two observers. These individuals might be members of a quality assurance department, or clinical nurses who have been trained in the use of the tool and whose status as practising nurses will enable their acceptance as peers by the group under review.

Making peer review work

The distinctive feature of peer review is that it involves each nurse judging the work of her peers and being judged herself by them. If the system is to have meaning it must be seen to be quite different from a management-imposed quality control system. The impetus to develop a system may come from management, the work of developing the system may be delegated to individuals or small groups, and only a few nurses may be actively involved at any one time, but the development must have the support and commitment of all the staff or it will not be true peer review.

The first requirement for successful peer review is that at least a majority of the staff involved perceive the need for and the value of peer review. This in turn requires a reasonable understanding of such issues as professionalism, accountability and responsibility. If a team of nurses are spontaneously considering peer review this in itself is probably indicative of a fairly advanced state of development. If the initiative comes from management or from one or two activists, these issues will have to be addressed before any further work is done.

Setting standards

Before any attempt at measurement of quality can be made a frame of reference must be established. The competencies required by the Nurses and Midwives Act, and the UKCC Code of Professional Conduct may provide a starting-point, as will locally-agreed philosophies of nursing and local policies. These issues have been dealt with in detail in another chapter but it is sufficient to emphasise here that, whatever standards and measuring tools are agreed upon they must be acceptable to the staff involved. It is probably better initially to keep things simple: as Brook *et al* (1976) point out, poor care usually comes from not doing known, easy things well.

Individual or collective practice?

The decision to apply peer review to the work of individual nurses or to the work of the team is one that must be made by the staff involved, influenced by their purpose in carrying out peer review, their clinical setting and their level of development. In areas such as the operating theatre, district nursing and health visiting, the labour suite, psychiatry, units practising primary nursing and any area where there is a clear responsibility placed on one nurse for a client or clients, individual peer review would seem to be appropriate. In any ward setting where primary nursing is not the chosen model, it would be more reasonable to review the work of the group collectively. The other area where individual practice review would be appropriate is in the educational setting as part of the process of assessment of the student.

Who should be the reviewers?

This topic has already been discussed at some length. The main point is, of course, that whoever it is should be acceptable to those being reviewed. If the results of the review are to be linked to promotion, salary awards or contract renewal, the reviewers must be acceptable to both the peer group and management. Distinctions must be made between professional qualifications and management grades. Can the staff nurse, charge nurse and director be considered to be peers, just because they have the same qualifications? Ciske *et al* argue strongly against the peer group being equated with the work group, when that includes nurses of different qualifications, such as enrolment and registration. These are all questions that must be thrashed out to the satisfaction of all the staff involved. In some systems of individual practice review the nurse is permitted to select her own reviewer. In other systems a consumer representative is included on the panel, although such a person could hardly be called a peer. One way around this problem would be to involve consumers in the initial standard-setting process.

Self-review

Anyone involved with student assessment or staff appraisal will know that most people are aware of their strengths and weaknesses and, given the opportunity, will be quite self-critical. Experienced assessors and appraisers will also know how much easier their job becomes once the individual has been allowed to give his account of himself. By the same token, whether individual or collective practice is being reviewed, those being reviewed should be encouraged to make their own assessment, either before the review takes place or before the results are reported. This self-review should include the identification of strengths as well as weaknesses.

Methods of review

Needless to say, whatever method of review is chosen, it should be acceptable to those using it and appropriate to the area of practice. Any of the published quality measurement tools may be used, or a unique system may be developed in-house. If the system requires outside observers trained in the use of the tool, and these individuals are not regarded as part of the peer group, the process should be seen as one of contracting, the staff group approaching the reviewers and requesting the review and then taking ownership of the resulting report and deciding for themselves how to use it.

In the case of review of individual practice the method may include, in addition to any observation of practice or chart audit, the presentation of a case study or piece of original work by the nurse concerned.

Handling the feedback

Peer review, like any other form of appraisal or assessment, should be a positive, constructive, creative experience for both reviewer and reviewed. There should be both affirmation and commendation of good practice and the identification of areas for growth and development. Where there is need for censure this should not be shirked, but criticism must be handled in a way which does not attack the personal integrity of the individual or cause a loss of self-esteem. One of the main advantages of peer review is that, as a member of the group, the reviewer feels a responsibility for the standards within the group, as well as knowing that the judge today will herself be judged tomorrow.

As has already been suggested, if there has been an honest self-review, the job of reporting back becomes much simpler. It is much easier to agree with a self-assessment of weakness, much nicer to be able to say 'it was not as bad as you expected', and much better to be able to confirm strengths and even amplify them. It is, in any case, of little use to tell someone about his faults if he has no insight and will not acknowledge them.

When providing feedback of this kind it is important to be able to give clear, specific examples of good and bad practice which can be related to the agreed standards or measuring tool. Just as peer review requires that the practitioner should be accountable for his practice, so the reviewer must be equally prepared to justify and defend his position.

Action plans

The most exciting part of peer review is the point at which the group or individual has thoroughly assimilated the review findings and can set objectives and plan courses of action based on the reviewers' report. Care should be taken not to attempt too much too quickly: objectives should be, as always, challenging but attainable. Contracting is a useful technique, either for the group or for individuals, and the help of outside consultants and other resources may be appropriate.

Problems

The biggest single problem that can afflict an undertaking such as peer review is lack of support and commitment from the staff involved. If the system is not valued or perceived to be necessary or helpful then it will founder.

A potential problem within the system is defensiveness on the part of those being reviewed. Peer review, by definition, requires a high degree of self-disclosure and risk-taking and it is natural for those involved to feel threatened. If the threat is too great, the natural reaction may be anger, hostility and denial, followed by a refusal to take part in any future reviews. Good preparation and self-review can help to reduce this risk, as can careful selection of the review team. If the reviewers are not perceived as true peers, but are seen as being removed from the clinical situation or lacking in appropriate specialist knowledge, it will be much easier for the staff to rationalise or deny the validity of the report.

Some theoretical considerations

It is intended in the next few paragraphs to develop some of the issues raised briefly, earlier in the chapter.

Most writers, nursing, medical and sociological, discuss peer review in terms of its relationship to professionalism. Typically, society recognises, that a particular service or occupation requires knowledge and expertise not accessible to the uninitiated. The authority and responsibility for the provision of the service is vested in the members of the profession and, in the words of Froebe & Bain (1976) there exists a 'social contract' between the profession and society, with peer review the accepted means of control and ensuring quality. The resulting 'professional monopoly' has come under severe criticism from writers such as Illich (1976) and others, and has been actively challenged in British society of late, particularly in the work of the legal profession.

The medical profession has always fought for and maintained its autonomy, placing great importance on self regulation and clinical freedom. Nursing, however, has been in rather a different position for, historically, it has its roots in service and has tended to be dependent on medicine. Nurses have allowed themselves to become part of an elaborate hierarchical bureaucracy, something which the classical professions have always avoided. Fisher (1983) refers to ' ... the tone of passivity that often pervades the profession.' and goes on to assert that nursing by its nature attracts people who 'profess qualities of dedication and devotion and who are service-orientated'. If peer review is to succeed in nursing there must be a change of attitude and an increased assertiveness. Development in this direction is of course hindered by the bureaucratic structure of health care: because most nurses work in hospitals, structural control is likely to exceed peer control.

Assuming that it is possible for nurses to develop professionally and achieve autonomy and self-regulation, a further dilemma must be faced. Peer review is based on the assumption that 'only nurses are competent to evaluate nursing care' (Froebe & Bain 1976). However, as Sidel (1976) argues, quality, on one level, is in the eye of the beholder. Definitions of quality made by members of a profession will reflect the values and opinions of the profession, which are not necessarily the same as those of the consumer. Sidel argues that a definition of quality should take into account those things that prevent the client from playing a role in health care systems, particularly feelings of powerlessness and intimidation by professionals.

There are encouraging signs that some British nurses are aware of such problems and are developing approaches to nursing that actively involve the patient in setting priorities and making decisions about his care. However, there is a long way to go before we can claim to have made real progress in areas such as communication skills and health education. Methods such as peer review are thus a double-edged sword. On one side, the development of accountability is encouraged and nurses are encouraged to break away from the domination of medicine and hierarchy. On the other, they are provided with the opportunity to fall into the very same pitfalls of professional monopoly for which medicine and the other classical professions have been so roundly condemned.

Nursing should be in a sense an 'antiprofession', seeking to recognise the patient's right to contribute to his own care and to restore independence rather than creating dependence. As long as this is clearly recognised, peer review can be a powerful tool, working for the mutual benefit of nurse and client.

References

Allbritten D Boland M Hubert P & Kiernan B (1982) Peer review: a practical guide. *Paediatric Nursing*, January/February, 31–32

Australian Hospital Association (1978) *Peer Review and Cost Containment – an Appraisal*. Health Service Monograph No. 1 SP/78

Beyers M & Phillips C (1979) *Nursing Management for Patient Care*. Boston: Little, Brown

Brook R H Williams K N & Avery A D (1976) Quality assurance today and tomorrow: forecast for the future. *Annals of Internal Medicine*, **85**, 809–817

Ciske K L Verhey C A & Ejan E C (1983) Improving peer relationships through contracting in primary nursing. *Journal of Nursing Administration*, February, 5–9

Cleland V S (1983) Taft-Hartley amended: Implications for nursing – the professional model. In Duespohl T A (ed) *Nursing in Transition*. Maryland: Aspen Systems Corporation

Fisher S M (1983) P S R O: Can it work in nursing. In Duespohl T A (ed) *Nursing in Transition*. Maryland: Aspen Systems Corporation

Froebe D J & Bain R J *Quality Assurance Programmes and Controls in Nursing*. St Louis: C V Mosby

Illich I (1976) *Limits to Medicine*. Harmondsworth: Penguin Books

Lamberton M Kee M & Adomanis A (1977) Peer Review in a family nurse clinician programme. *Nursing Outlook*, **25**, January

Maas M & Jacox A K (1977) *Guidelines for Nurse Autonomy/Patient Welfare*. New York: Appleton-Century-Crofts

Mullins A C Colavecchio R E Tescher B E (1979) Peer review: a model for professional accountability. *Journal of Nursing Administration*, December, 25–30

O'Loughlin E L Kaulbach D (1981) Peer review: a perspective for performance appraisal. *Journal of Nursing Administration*, September, 22–27

Passos J A (1973) Accountability: myth or mandate. *Journal of Nursing Administration*, **3**(3), 17–22

Ramphal M (1974) Peer review. *American Journal of Nursing*, 64

Sidel V W (1976) Quality for whom? The effects of professional responsibility for quality of health care on equity. *Bulletin of the New York Academy of Medicine*, **52**, 164–176

3
Quality of Patient Care Scale

ANNE WILES

The Quality Patient Care Scale (Qualpacs) was designed to measure the standard of nursing received by a patient, or a group of patients. Much of the content and structure of this scale has been derived from the Slater Nursing Performance Rating Scale. The Slater (1967) scale evaluates the competence of an individual nurse as she is observed giving care to her patients. Her performance is measured against a given standard, which is provided by the scale. It can be used in any environment where nurses work with clients, and over any length of time in excess of two and a half hours.

As the Slater scale proved to be both effective and practicable in its use, it was surmised that a similar format could be used to measure the quality of care received by patients.

Development of QUALPACS

The development of Qualpacs was undertaken at Wayne State University, where some of the work associated with the Slater scale was also done. Many of the same personnel contributed to each project.

The Slater scale consists of 84 items, all of which were considered pertinent to the performance of a nurse. It was found that many of these items could also apply to the care received by a patient, with some adjustment to the wording. However, some items were excluded as being unsuitable, while other dimensions of care were included through the addition of completely new items.

The new scale was tested in three Detroit hospitals before being distributed throughout the United States of America. The testing, and subsequent results, appeared to indicate that the scale was both usable and reliable. Hospitals and

25

nursing homes found that it drew attention to the differences and deficiencies in care, and that it provided baseline data for improvement programmes.

The Qualpacs scale, and the instructions for its use, was published in 1974 (Wandelt & Ager 1974) and a copy of this scale can be found at the end of this chapter.

Qualpacs will give a measurement of the quality of care provided by a ward or unit, but not that which is given by a particular nurse. Experienced assessors evaluate the nursing received by a number of a ward's patients, and that standard is then regarded as a reflection of the care to all the clients of that ward.

It is the content, or process, of nursing which is scrutinised. This is done through direct observation of care, and by obtaining evidence of actions from the nursing records. The assessors allocate a score to every observable action which they judge to be part of the nursing of their selected patients. These actions may take the form of direct care, occurring during interactions between a patient and his nurse, or they may be performed on behalf of the patient. The latter category includes the teaching of nursing skills to a relative or giving information to other professional workers.

The QUALPACS schedule

The content of nursing covers a very wide range of activities: for the purpose of this scale, these activities have been analysed, and organised into 68 elements of care. These elements, or items, have then been classified under six broad headings which are described by the authors as follows (the number of items ascribed to each of the classifications is also given):

1. *Psychosocial: individual*
   Actions directed toward meeting psychosocial needs of individual patients
   15 items

2. *Psychosocial: group*
   Actions directed toward meeting psychosocial needs of patients as members of a group
   8 items

3. *Physical*
   Actions directed toward meeting the physical needs of patients
   15 items

4. *General*
   Actions that may be directed toward meeting either psychosocial or physical needs of the patient, or both at the same time
   15 items

5. *Communication*
   Communication on behalf of the patient
   8 items

6. *Professional Implications*
   Care given to patients reflects initiative and responsibility indicative of professional expectations
   7 items

   Total = 68 items

The items are written as statements concerning the standard of care received by a patient: for example, the item 'Patient receives nurse's full attention' is classified under the heading 'Psychosocial: individual', while the item 'Patient is encouraged to observe appropriate rest and exercise' can be found under 'Physical' needs of the patient. An assessor is required to judge the extent to which she can agree with the statements.

To help an observer in making her decisions, the authors have provided examples of the kind of actions which can lead to a judgement about a particular item of care. These examples are termed 'cues'. They can help an assessor to select the most appropriate item when recording an observed action, and can remind assessors about the sorts of activities which can be evaluated. The full list of the cues for the 68 items can be obtained from Wandelt & Ager (1974) but, as an example, the cues provided for the item 'Patient receives nurse's full attention' are as follows:

(a) patient is appropriately responded to, verbally and non-verbally, without being asked to repeat phrases;
(b) staff assumes positions that will aid in observation and communication with the patient;
(c) conversation of staff is restricted to patient who is receiving care;
(d) the infant is looked at and talked to as he receives a bottle feed;
(e) questions are posed which encourage patient to express feelings;
(f) evidence is given by staff of anticipation of projected needs of patient.

These cues are not intended to be a comprehensive list of actions, but are suggestions. An assessor may modify a cue to suit a particular environment, make additions, or construct a personal list of cues. These alterations do not affect the scale as it is the items which are scored, not the cues. The cues are simply illustrations of the kind of nurse actions which can be attributed to each of the items. It is recommended that assessors should read through their cues just before commencing a period of observation, to refresh the memory, and should refer to them as necessary during the assessment.

Using the tool

When using Qualpacs to evaluate the care provided by a ward, it is essential that at least two assessors should collect the data. This reduces the risk of observer bias, as it is probable that most nurses will have some personal belief regarding the relative importance of some aspects of care. These differences should be cancelled out when the observations and scores of two or more assessors are combined.

The evaluation may also provide a more realistic impression of a ward if assessments take place at various times of the day and night and, perhaps, on different days of the week.

As a guide to the number of observation periods required, it is recommended that the care received by 15 per cent or 5 of the patients, whichever is the higher number, should be assessed. The number of patients who may be observed at any one time depends upon the layout of the ward, and the level of care required by the patients. The assessors should use their own judgement when deciding whether to watch just one patient, or a small group.

Although Wandelt & Ager (1974) believe than an experienced assessor can work alone, it may be more advantageous for two observers to watch the same incidents. A criticism or recommendation may be considered more valid if it is made by two independent witnesses.

Before the evaluation of a ward commences, the person who has requested the assessment should make sure that the nursing staff know what to expect. It could be argued that this knowledge would alter the behaviour of the nurses but it seems that the presence of observers is soon forgotten, and that nurses quickly become accustomed to being watched. The staff should be asked to allocate and carry out their nursing care in their usual way, but be prepared to provide the visitors with information. On arrival in the ward, the observers should first select their patient or patients. Complete random selection is not feasible, so the assessors should choose a patient, or number of patients, who are representative of the ward's clients. If more than one patient is to be observed, it must be possible to watch them simultaneously without undue difficulty.

The permission of the selected patients should be sought, after they have been informed about the procedure. They need to know that the visitors are nurses who will be watching their own nurses. It is also wise to inform all other patients and visitors who can see what is happening. This can help in avoiding misunderstandings and anxieties.

When the patients have been selected and the assessors introduced to all concerned, the collection of data is commenced. A verbal report is obtained from a nurse who is responsible for the chosen patients. If it is appropriate, the assessors may listen to the change-of-shift report, otherwise they should ask for the necessary information. The nursing records are then consulted.

Using all the information available to them, the assessors should construct their own outline care plan for their patient, or patients. This plan will give an indication of the actions which the observers expect to see, and is dependent upon their professional knowledge and judgement.

When the assessors have established the needs of their patients, they should be ready to start their observation. They should find an unobtrusive position, but one which will allow them to both see and hear their selected patients. A two-hour period of direct observation follows.

During this time, the assessors take the role of non-participant observers. They should not communicate with the patients, relatives or any member of staff, and everyone should be warned that they are not to be engaged in conversation, or even in non-verbal exchanges. They should make no contribution to nursing care. This may prove difficult, as observers may have to resist a response to a patient's obvious need. But they should always remember that any interventions on their part will alter the care received by the patient.

The only circumstances under which the observers are allowed, or obliged, to intervene are those which are dangerous to the patient. An observer would not watch while a patient fell out of bed, and should always alert the ward staff to any serious change in a patient's condition; otherwise, she should simply take note of all that occurs, or does not occur. It is probably inadvisable for assessors to wear a nurse's uniform, as this invites requests for assistance. Their own personal clothing seems to be suitable, although some observers may prefer to add a white laboratory coat.

It is permissible for assessors to enter behind screens to watch some aspect of care, provided that the patient has no objection. Knowing that the observers are nurses, patients do not seem to mind this intrusion but it is obviously necessary to use sensitivity in determining the extent of the direct observation, and to respect their right to privacy. A surprising amount of information can be gained through attentive listening, supplemented by a discreet peep behind the curtains.

Each observer should have a copy of the Qualpacs scale and her list of cues. She will record all her observations on the same one copy, even if she is watching care being given to several patients.

As each interaction between a nurse and a selected patient commences, the observer will mentally analyse the nurse's actions. She will break these down into parts, and assign each part to one of the 68 items. For example, a nurse may approach a patient to offer him a drink. The observer may note the manner in which she addresses the patient, the degree of attention the patient receives, the skill with which the patient is encouraged to drink, and any recording of the incident. Such an interaction could result in parts of the nurse's actions being assigned to items 1, 3, 6, 13, 24, 26, 31, 44, 49, 51, and 56, or even more, depending upon the complexity and content. If an observer has a problem in selecting the most appropriate item for a particular action, she may find the answer in her cue list.

The items to which the actions have been attributed must then be scored, according to the standard to which they were performed. The scale allows an item to be rated as 'best care', 'between', 'average care', 'between' or 'poorest care' by placing a mark in the appropriate column (Fig. 3.1).

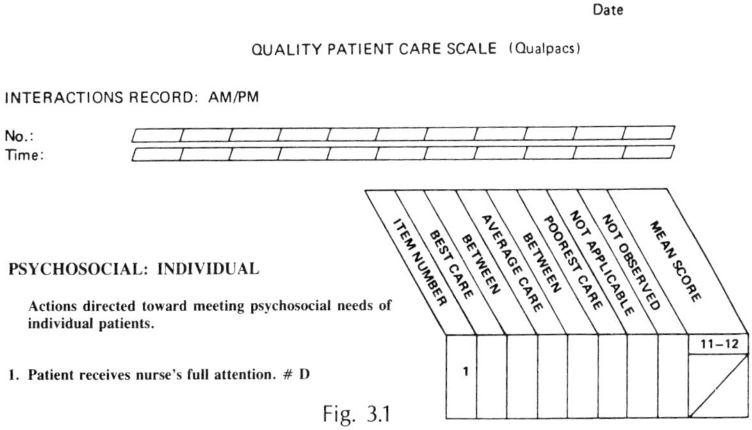

Fig. 3.1

The observer who has watched a nurse offer a drink to a patient may believe that the kindness and attention shown to the patient was an average standard, while the encouragement to drink was a little less well done. She may note that there was no allowance for the patient's personal preferences or abilities.

She would, therefore, mark items 1, 3, 6, and 26 as 'average care', items 31 and 44 as 'poorest care', and items 13 and 24 in the 'between' average and poorest care column (Fig. 3.2).

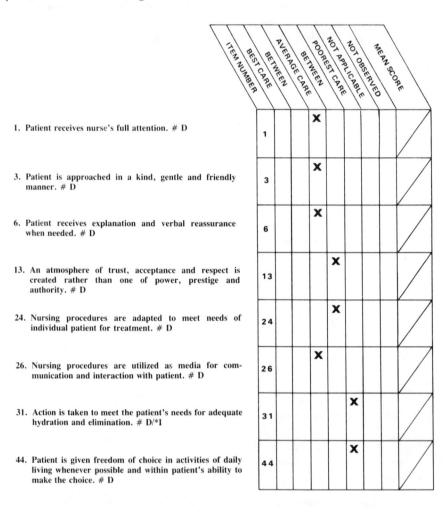

Fig. 3.2

An interaction is considered to be finished when there is some interruption in the communication between the patient and the nurse. The nurse may leave the room, or she may turn her attention to another person. Even if the same nurse soon returns to the patient, this is considered to be another interaction, and the analysis and scoring commences afresh.

The number and commencing time of each interaction is recorded at the top of the scale. This may help in identifying busy periods, and the sequence and timing of nursing care.

As further interactions take place, several scores will accumulate against some of the items. For instance, any communication between patient and nurse must result in some appraisal of the attention and kindness displayed. An item must be scored each time it is considered to be part of a new interaction, even if the nurse and the quality of her care both remain the same (Fig. 3.3).

Item	Item Number	Best Care	Between	Average Care	Between	Poorest Care	Not Applicable	Not Observed	Mean Score
1. Patient receives nurse's full attention. # D	1	X	X	X X	X	X			
3. Patient is approached in a kind, gentle and friendly manner. # D	3	X	X	X X	X X				
6. Patient receives explanation and verbal reassurance when needed. # D	6	X		X X		X			
13. An atmosphere of trust, acceptance and respect is created rather than one of power, prestige and authority. # D	13	X		X X	X	X			
24. Nursing procedures are adapted to meet needs of individual patient for treatment. # D	24	X		X	X				
26. Nursing procedures are utilized as media for communication and interaction with patient. # D	26	X		X X	X				
31. Action is taken to meet the patient's needs for adequate hydration and elimination. # D/*I	31			X		X			
44. Patient is given freedom of choice in activities of daily living whenever possible and within patient's ability to make the choice. # D	44		X	X		X			

Fig. 3.3

When she is judging the quality of observed care to be best, average or poor, it is obviously necessary for an assessor to have some standard in mind. This standard should be the care which can be expected of a first-level staff nurse. This person would be a registered nurse who is employed to meet the nursing needs of the patients of that ward or unit. She would have appropriate education for her job, including any necessary post-basic course, but no additional experience or qualifications. All observed nursing actions should be measured against this standard.

It is true that this is a very broad and general concept, yet the testing of this scale has shown that there is a high level of agreement between experienced nurses on what they expect of such a nurse.

It could also be said that this is not a fair measurement, as much direct care is provided by untrained nurses or those in training. But if a flexible standard was used, which could be altered according to the education and experience of a nurse, the final score would not have the same meaning. With a fixed standard it is possible to confirm or refute expectations regarding differences in the quality of care given by various groups or grades of nurses.

This scale focuses on the care received by patients. A patient is entitled to a certain standard of nursing, which may be defined as that which he would receive from a registered nurse. If his care is poorer in quality owing to his nurse's lack of knowledge or skill, surely this should be regarded as a fault in the organisation of nursing, not an inevitability. The use of a fixed standard should highlight these deficits, while a flexible standard might hide them.

If it is useful to measure the influence of education or experience upon a nurse's performance, then it is necessary to identify the grade of nurse who is responsible for each action. This is done by using symbols when recording scores against the items. For example, S may be used to represent a ward sister, R used for a registered nurse, L for a learner, and so on (Fig. 3.4).

These symbols should be predetermined by an assessor, and noted on the form. She may use any code she chooses, a personal selection probably being easier for her to remember and to use quickly without difficulty. The names of the nurses should not be recorded on the form. This means that the nursing staff can be assured of anonymity, although they can be identified by status.

The assessors will make appropriate recordings on the scale whenever they observe actions which they believe to be part of the nursing of their patients. If a relative gives care, this should also be scored if it is planned or supervised by one of the nurses.

If she wishes, an observer may record a number against each symbol, to correspond with the number of the interaction. This would allow a more detailed analysis of the content of each interaction at a later time. It may also be easier for an observer to check her entries if she is interrupted or becomes very busy (Fig. 3.5).

It is difficult to predict the events which may occur during an observation period. For instance, a patient may move to another environment, such as a day room or x-ray department. If it is at all possible, the assessor should remain with the patient and continue to rate his care.

The assessor may also find that she is unable to keep up with the events that are happening. Interactions may occur in very quick succession or, if more than one patient is being observed, two or several interactions may take place simultaneously. There are various ways to handle this situation.

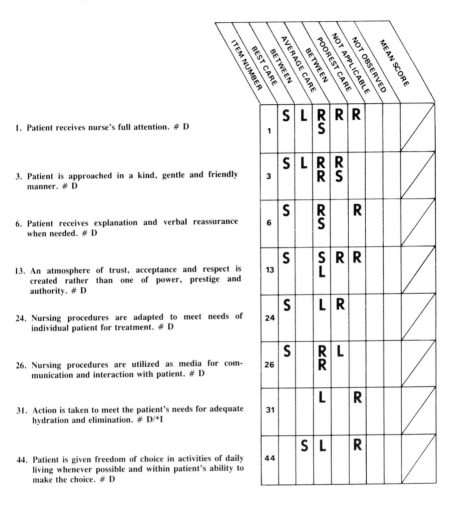

Fig. 3.4

If two assessors are present, they may agree to watch different patients, or different nurses interacting with the same patient. An assessor who is alone may decide to omit recording a second interaction until she has completed the first, or she may abandon the first incident and move on to the second. Alternatively, she could make reminder notes of the events and use these to score the items at a later time. Under these circumstances it is useful to continue recording the numbers and times of the interactions, so that the sequence may be more easily recalled.

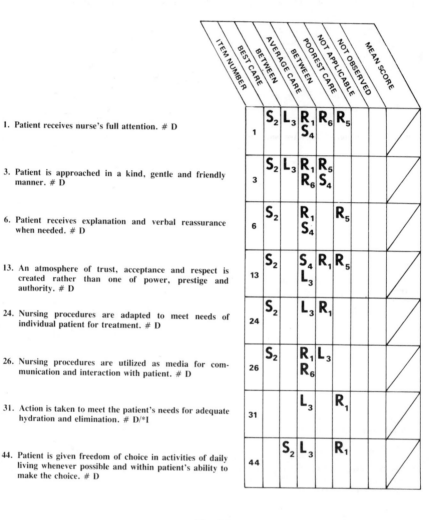

Fig. 3.5

The direct observation should cease after two hours. The assessors will then look for indirect evidence of care by consulting the records and charts. This evidence is also scored, using the same fixed standard. Where there is no available information regarding the status of the nurse, the symbol X should be used to record the score.

All the items will be reviewed by the assessors before they leave the ward. They may wish to add further scores to some of the items, based on recalled observations but some, or perhaps many, of the items will have received no scores.

The assessor must decide whether an unscored item is relevant to her patient. If it is not, then it is marked with an X in the 'not applicable' column. However, if the item is pertinent to the patient, but no actions related to it were seen during the observation period, the assessor must decide whether this omission was reasonable. She may seek further information by questioning the nurses or from the records. Her own care plan should prove useful at this time, as it indicates the assessor's initial expectations.

If she is led to believe that some aspect of care was scheduled for another time, or that the need did not arise during the given period, she should record this fact by placing an X in the 'not observed' column. But if care related to an item was not provided, although it was needed and could be expected, then this is always regarded to be 'poorest care'. These omissions are recorded in the appropriate column, using X as the symbol (Fig. 3.6).

Item	Item Number	Best Care	Between	Average Care	Between	Poorest Care	Not Applicable	Not Observed	Mean Score
10. The rejecting or demanding patient continues to receive acceptance. # D/*I	10						X		
15. The unconscious or nonoriented patient is cared for with the same respectful manner as the conscious patient. # D	15							X	
18. Patient receives encouragement to participate in or to plan for the group's daily activities. # D	18								X
64. Changes in care and care plans reflect continuous evaluation of results of nursing care. # D/*I	64						X		

Fig. 3.6

To help an assessor in making these decisions, each item on the scale is marked D (direct), *I (indirect) or both. This is to show whether an item can only be evaluated through direct observation, of if indirect methods are more appropriate, or that either mode may be used.

When the scale has been checked, every item should have at least one symbol recorded against it. It has been estimated that one observation period requires the assessors to spend three hours in a ward or unit. But their work is not finished until the mean score has been calculated. The arithmetic, and the comparisons between the findings of different assessors, should take place when the observers have left the ward.

The first step in calculating a total mean score is to find the mean score of each item. Every entry against an item is awarded a value on a five-point scale, from 5 for 'best care', through 3 for 'average care' to 1 for 'poorest care'. These figures are added together to give a total score for the item. This number is recorded above and to the left of the diagonal line in the 'mean score' column (Fig. 3.7).

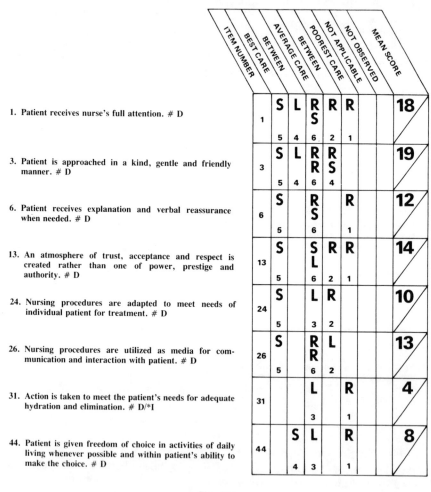

Fig. 3.7

This total score is then divided by the number of entries made against that item, giving a mean score for the item. This number is recorded below and to the right of the diagonal line (Fig. 3.8).

This procedure is repeated for each of the 68 items, with those items which were rated as 'not applicable' or 'not observed' receiving no score.

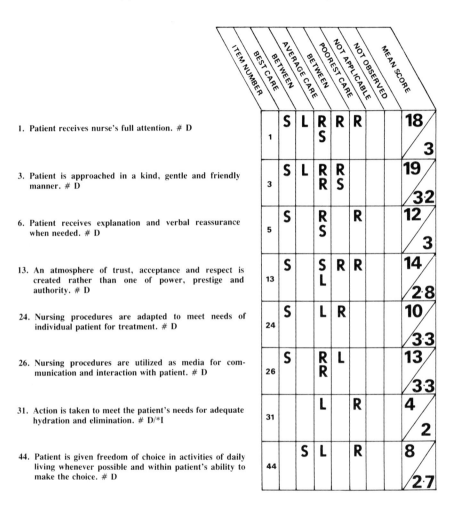

Fig. 3.8

The total mean score provides an overall measurement of the quality of care received by the observed patients. This is found by adding all the item means together, and dividing this figure by the number of items which received a score. 'Not applicable' and 'not observed' items are excluded from these calculations. These figures are recorded at the end of the scale (Fig. 3.9).

The mean scores of each of the areas can then be calculated in a similar manner. The mean scores of each of the items within an area are added together, and this total is divided by the number of items which received a score. These figures are recorded at the end of each subsection (Fig. 3.10).

66. Assigned staff keep informed of the patient's condition and whereabouts. # D

67. Care given the patient reflects flexibility in rules and regulations as indicated by individual patient needs. # D/*I

68. Organization and management of nursing activities reflect due consideration for patient needs. # D/*I

66	S R		R			9 / 3
67	L R S R					11 / 2·8
68	R L S		R			11 / 2·8

AREA VI MEAN

Sum of Item Means   **147·8**
Number of Items Rated   **46**

Mean of Item Means   **3·2**

Fig. 3.9

66. Assigned staff keep informed of the patient's condition and whereabouts. # D

67. Care given the patient reflects flexibility in rules and regulations as indicated by individual patient needs. # D/*I

68. Organization and management of nursing activities reflect due consideration for patient needs. # D/*I

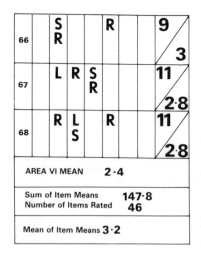

AREA VI MEAN   **2·4**

Sum of Item Means   **147·8**
Number of Items Rated   **46**

Mean of Item Means **3·2**

Fig. 3.10

It is not arithmetically correct to use the mean scores of the area subsections to calculate the total mean score. This may only be done by adding all the item means together, and dividing this number by the number of items scored.

Two observers who have worked together on an assessment should take the opportunity to discuss their findings, and to compare their scores. This tends to increase their awareness and their confidence in their own judgement.

Unless an observation period is simply a learning exercise for prospective assessors, it is probable that a report is required. The person who has requested the assessment should receive the report. She may be a manager but, ideally, she should be the leader of the clinical team of that ward or unit.

The report should give the overall mean score, and a general impression of the quality of the care which was observed. The scores for the subsections are also given, with examples of the actions which led to these scores. It is important that examples of both good and bad care are provided, and that selected incidents are described without mentioning names. The ward staff should remain anonymous, and as unidentifiable as is possible.

If more than one period of observation has taken place, the scores and impressions from all the assessments should be combined to give a composite report. The final scores will be calculated by finding the means of the total scores, and those of the subsections.

These scores should be compared with any previous assessments, so that improvements or other changes are shown. It is important that strengths, as well as weaknesses, are indicated. Otherwise, an assessment can be a most demoralising process for the ward staff.

The points which require improvement should be stated explicitly, with no scope for misunderstandings. Recommendations can be made, if this is thought to be necessary. These can ask for attention to the educational needs of the staff, or for changes in ward management, services or staffing complement. If the assessment was requested for a specific purpose, ie. before altering the ratio of trained to untrained staff, these points should be especially noted and comments made.

It is also necessary to comment on any unusual incident, or any factor which could affect the standard of care. This would include any emergency, sickness amongst the staff, or multiple ward rounds which occupied a lot of nursing time.

If the results are poor, the assessors can ask for improvements to be made within a given period. They can also make an appointment for a further assessment. This should take place after three months, six months or any timespan which seems appropriate to the situation.

If the assessors are seriously concerned about the standard of care provided by a ward, they can ask for the report to be taken to the nurse manager. They will not normally do this themselves, unless the clinical nurse did not fulfil the request. (This, of course, supposes that the clinical nurse asked for the assessment to take place.)

When the report is sent to the ward, the staff should be given the opportunity to ask for a meeting with the assessors. If they accept the report as being valid, and agree with the findings and recommendations, this may not be necessary. But, sometimes, clarification and discussion can prove very useful.

In summary, the assessors' report to the nursing staff should include the following information:

1   mean score for the observed care;
2   the assessors' overall impression of the care;
3   mean scores recorded for the subsections;
4   good points, with examples;
6   points for improvement, with examples;
7   comparison with the report from any previous assessment;
8   suggestions and recommendations for change.

Who should act as assessors

If the report and recommendations are to be considered valid, it is necessary for the assessors to appear credible to the ward staff: they must be regarded as being suitably qualified to evaluate the care given by their colleagues. It is therefore important that the criteria for their selection should be carefully established. Some of the points for consideration are given as follows, but experience may result in other items being added to this list.

(a)   Adequate clinical experience is an obvious essential requirement. Perhaps a minimum of three or four years of post-registration practice should be considered acceptable. This practice should have involved the delivery of direct patient care.

(b)   A good professional reputation is required. So, although it is probably most suitable for self-selection to be the usual means of recruitment, the assessors must possess high clinical nursing standards. The standards of an individual may be ascertained through references from managers or teachers, or perhaps the use of the Slater scale would provide assurance of a nurse's competence.

(c)   The ward staff will need to believe that an assessor is familiar with current nursing practices, and that she has recently experienced the stresses of clinical work. It could be said that all assessors need to be clinically active, the extent of their involvement being exactly defined. If the acceptable minimum amount of clinical contact with patients is predetermined, eg. one day per week on a regular basis, it will be possible for managers, teachers and part-time staff to decide upon their own eligibility.

(d)   The assessors should be thoroughly familiar with the scale. They will need to be quick and confident in making decisions and recordings, and will therefore require both tuition and practice in the use of the tool before embarking on an assessment.

The setting-up of a Qualpacs team as part of a quality control programme is dependent upon the recruitment of an adequate number of interested, suitable and well-prepared nurses. The number of assessors should be sufficient easily to meet the needs of the clinical areas. If their number is too low, an undue burden will be placed upon the few who are available. It is also inevitable that some assessments will be postponed. This is likely to lead to a loss of enthusiasm, both amongst the assessors and those members of the clinical staff who want to be assessed.

Recruitment to a team of Qualpacs assessors should be based on self-selection, as interest and enthusiasm are vital. Publicity plays an important role at this stage, as potential assessors need to know that they are required, and exactly what this commitment would mean. The criteria for eligibility should be made quite clear.

At first, nurses may be reticent about volunteering for an unfamiliar role but, as interest in quality control increases and Qualpacs assessments are seen to take place within clinical areas, more members of staff should elect to become involved.

It is probably most suitable for potential assessors to learn about Qualpacs in the context of a workshop or small learning group. This should allow anxieties to be expressed, and experiences and ideas to be shared. The participants in these workshops could include some nurses, such as managers or teachers, who are ineligible to become assessors but need to understand the uses and benefits of the tool.

In order that the group may develop some general understanding of quality assurance, the subject can be introduced from a wider perspective. An exploration of the aims of a quality control programme and the possible approaches, can lead on to consideration of the available data and methods. The ensuing detailed examination of the Qualpacs scale could then be undertaken with some appreciation of the place of this tool within a comprehensive programme.

During the workshop, the learning group should be given the opportunity to practice using the scale. This exercise should provide insight into the practicalities, and increase individual confidence. Real-life clinical situations are required, with two or three nurses observing the same patient. At this stage, one patient is sufficient, as it is difficult for those who are unfamiliar with the scale to cope with many interactions. The identification of items appears to present the most difficulty, with learners tending to spend much time in searching for the most appropriate classification for an observation.

Following this observation period, the group can score their recorded items. A comparison of the results obtained by pairs of observers should reveal similarities. If this is not the case, a detailed comparison of events and observations should show why these differences have occurred.

Members of the group may express surprise that their scores accurately reflect their impressions of the observed care. This may be particularly notable where the clinical area was markedly different from a nurse's usual place of work. It does, in fact, appear to be easier for a nurse to be objective when she is faced with an unfamiliar environment, and very difficult, if not impossible, for her to evaluate the care given by friends or colleagues. The nature of the observer's clinical experience does not appear to be important. The experienced nurse can distinguish between good and bad practice, and she has the option of asking the ward staff for clarification of any point. She is also obliged to quote specific incidents when writing her report. It is therefore possible for a community nurse to evaluate the work of an intensive care unit, or an accident department nurse to assess the care given by nurses to the elderly sick.

Following this initial learning experience, those nurses who wish to become

Qualpacs assessors will require further practice. Group members can arrange this amongst themselves, as their individual requirements will differ. However, a further meeting, or meetings, for the whole group will provide essential peer support, and an opportunity for the discussion of experiences, difficulties and successes.

A nurse can only decide for herself that she is ready to become an assessor. She must feel satisfied that she is thoroughly conversant with the scale, and confident that she can quickly assign and record her observations. She may then inform the quality assurance co-ordinator, who should accept her as an assessor provided that she meets the established criteria.

The quality assurance co-ordinator

If a nursing service is to be offered the opportunity to have the process of nursing evaluated through Qualpacs, it is probably necessary for someone to be designated quality assurance co-ordinator. This person's role would reflect the service which is offered, but may include some of the following functions:

1   maintaining an up-to-date list of assessors
2   recruiting assessors
3   matching suitable, available assessors to requests for evaluation
4   providing secretarial services for the typing of reports
5   filing assessment forms and copies of reports
6   producing statistics and progress reports
7   contributing to the education of assessors

Any consideration of the role of this person must involve the clarification of several vital issues. The purpose of the programme should be established, and decisions made regarding the fate and availability of the reports. If the use of Qualpacs is seen as a management tool, the requests for assessment may be received from nurse managers, who will be given the report and could use the results to monitor staff performance. If, however, Qualpacs is only to be available for peer review, then requests must be made by clinical nurses, who will use the report to measure their own standards. Although copies of the reports should be kept by the co-ordinator, these should not be made available to managers unless this was previously agreed. The report would only be discussed with a manager under the circumstances which have previously been described. It is also necessary to make decisions regarding the nature and amount of the information to be revealed if a general progress report on the service is required.

In addition to these matters of policy, a hospital or health authority will need to consider the financial implications of this service. Each observation period will require three hours plus travelling time. Extra time should be allowed for discussion, collation of results and writing the report. As two observers work together, this time allowance should be doubled. This figure should give some indication of the cost of evaluating the care given by one ward or unit.

There is also the training period to be taken into account. Prospective assessors need two days to attend a workshop, and further time to practice using the tool. At least one teacher should be available to organise and lead the workshops, and to attend the follow-up meetings.

With the additional cost of the programme co-ordinator, secretarial help and stationery, it can be seen that the implementation of this service will not be cheap. However, no quality assurance system is without cost, and the expense may appear more justifiable when it is weighed against the possible benefits of such a programme.

The benefits of QUALPACS

The use of Qualpacs will provide clinical nurses with an evaluation of their performance. This knowledge may create an awareness which could lead to changes in practice. The need for change can be identified, specific goals can be set, and progress can be monitored by subsequent reports. Positive evaluations can provide encouragement, and the emphasis on group performance should increase both the cohesion and the performance of the nursing team.

It is, however, not only the observed who benefit from this system. The process of observing the experience of clients appears to increase the sensitivity of nurses. Observers have reported a heightened awareness of the needs of patients, with a resultant examination of their own standards.

It would seem that the experience of observing the process of nursing can be valuable for all nurses, including students. The opportunity to watch the expert practitioner, whilst using the Qualpacs scale as a framework, could aid the nursing student in gaining knowledge of the content of nursing. It could also help her to appreciate the range of possible responses to a given situation, and have a beneficial effect on her observation skills.

There are other ways in which Qualpacs may be useful in nurse education. The scale can provide information about nursing standards when wards are being selected as training areas and it can help to identify needs for continuing education, and to assess the efficacy of any educational programme.

The nurse researcher can use Qualpacs to compare the quality of care provided in different settings, or before and after an intervention. It could also be incorporated into an action research project, or help to provide the answers to questions about such issues as the organisation of nursing or the most appropriate mix of staff for a unit.

The periodic assessment of nursing standards may provide information for nurse managers. The need for resources, or their most effective use, may be identified, but most benefit to managers should arise from the knowledge that nursing practice is constantly under review.

An examination of the process of nursing may give some indication of the required structure, and the likely outcomes of care. Qualpacs can be criticised for the subjective nature of the tool, it being true that the use of the scale relies on the professional judgement of the assessors but this fact does not necessarily invalidate the method. Experienced nurses appear to agree about those actions which constitute 'good' or 'bad' care. If those actions can be recognised on observation, and a framework provided for their documentation, this expertise may be used to good effect as part of a comprehensive quality assurance programme.

References

Wandelt M A & Stewart D S (1975) *Slater Nursing Competency Rating Scale*. New York: Appleton-Century-Crofts

Wandelt M & Ager J (1974) *Quality Patient Care Scale*. New York: Appleton-Century-Crofts

4

Phaneuf's Nursing Audit

SUE BRADSHAW

Auditing of nursing records may be used concurrently or retrospectively, the basic principles being that a clear set of questions about care are posed and answers are sought from the records. The assumption is, therefore, that the records will faithfully represent the care given.

Phaneuf (1976) describes an audit schedule which is process-orientated, appraises the nursing process as it is reflected in the patients' records, and is a retrospective method of quality assurance. The audit schedule used by the auditors, utilises the functions of nursing listed by Lesnik & Anderson (1955):

1   The application and execution of the doctor's legal orders.
2   The observation of symptoms and reactions.
3   Supervision of the patients.
4   Supervision of those participating in care.
5   Reporting and recording.
6   The application of nursing procedures and techniques.
7   The promotion of health by directing and teaching.

From these seven functions, Phaneuf (1976) identifies 50 components to help auditors to evaluate the quality of nursing by 'focusing their attention on the patient rather than on the nursing specialities of the nurses who administer care' (Marrinner, 1979). The 50 components are stated in terms of actions by nurses in relation to the patient, and in the form of questions to be answered by the auditors as they review the patient's record.

In implementing audit as a method of quality assurance, the setting up of a nursing audit committee is recommended to serve as the 'professional nursing conscience of the agency concerned through its monthly performance of audits'. The committee should have at least five members, and each member should possess clinical competence, commitment to clinical nursing, and interest in quality control and an ability to work in a group. It is suggested that each member should review no more than ten patients each month, and that an auditor will be able to carry out a single audit in approximately 15 minutes when skill in using the method is acquired. If the number of discharges per month is less than 50, all may be audited, but when larger numbers are involved, patients may be selected so that 10 per cent of discharges are reviewed.

The instrument constructed for the use of auditors to evaluate systematically the care given as recorded in the records comprises three parts. Part one refers to the setting, and two separate formats are presented by Phaneuf – one specifically for hospital or nursing home care, and the other for community-based care. Phaneuf recommends that this section be completed by a member of the clerical staff as its completion does not demand nursing judgement. The items in it are not scored, although they may be referred to in the later parts of the audit.

Part two is the chart review schedule, and comprises the 50 components derived from the seven nursing functions outlined previously and posed in terms of questions to be answered by the auditors. In answering each question, provision is made for the auditor to respond with 'uncertain' and, in some items, 'does not apply'. The audit committee decides on what criteria they will accept as having met the requirements of each component. After completion of part two, the reply on each question is scored, and the score is then weighted according to the relative importance assigned to the component concerned. Phaneuf maintains that the weighting system has been derived from extensive testing of the instrument.

The final audit score is arrived at by multiplying the total score of individual component scores by a value determined by the 'does not apply' responses, and is entered on part three of the audit document. The final, numerical audit score is equated with one of five descriptive statements:

$$
\begin{aligned}
161 - 200 &= \text{excellent} \\
121 - 160 &= \text{good} \\
81 - 120 &= \text{incomplete} \\
41 - 80 &= \text{poor} \\
0 - 40 &= \text{unsafe}
\end{aligned}
$$

To use the Audit Chart effectively, it is important that the auditors discuss the seven nursing functions, the 50 subcomponents, and the definitions, followed by group examination of a single chart which reflects a total period of care not exceeding two weeks in length. Shorter charts are initially more difficult to audit, because the nursing process is ordinarily adapted to this time span of service. Longer stays yield discussion that is over-long for the purpose of practice definitions to 50 items.

The purpose of this exercise is to reach majority agreement on each of the 50 items. After discussion of evidence on some items, there is likely to be concensus; on others, there will be marked differences in judgement. Movement towards agreement is essential before auditing can begin.

The nursing audit of patient records has been widely criticised as a method of quality assurance. Hegyvary & Haussman (1976) purport that it only serves to improve documentation, not nursing care, and Mayers *et al* (1977) see its major fault as being its assumption that what is done is documented, and what is documented is done. Phaneuf (1976) suggests that good documentation leads to good nursing, but Jelinek *et al* (1974) argue that nurses soon learn how to document in a way which favourably influences the audit results, without necessarily changing the delivery of nursing. Despite the arguments, nursing audit may be useful as part of, but not necessarily as the total means of, a quality assurance programme if the records in use are accurate records of care. Records in current use in most British nursing situations are not likely to be suitable (Lelean 1973). In units where nursing records follow a nursing process approach, nursing audit may be a feasible and desirable component of an effort to evaluate the quality of nursing.

Using Phaneuf's nursing audit

Experience in using Phaneuf's method for auditing nursing notes was first gained as part of a training package. Notes were supplied by trainee auditors from their units and were audited in their own time and in their own environment. This proved to be interesting, although rather depressing, as most of the auditors became aware of the inadequacy of their own record-keeping. The training sessions provided them with the opportunity to assess the problems they were likely to encounter when providing the service in the clinical situation. Since the initial training of auditors and Qualpac assessors they have met together as a team and have agreed that only those with a defined clinical content in their work will be eligible to undertake assessments. This will preserve the credibility of the audit and auditors: it may also result in some changes in the audit team.

Quality Assurance Assessments are arranged by the co-ordinator of the team who, coincidentally, is also an auditor. The request originates from a clinical nurse in respect of her own ward or unit, no requests being accepted from nurse managers. The demand for assessments has been sufficiently great to create a waiting list which indicates the interest generated within the wards. So far they have included two very specialised units, acute medical and surgical wards and community hospitals. In some instances the nurses have requested information about the procedure, the feedback and the implication for practice before committing themselves while others appear happy to take the plunge. Although Phaneuf's tool lends itself to use with records kept by community nurses, no requests have been received to date; however, one group of district nurses has asked for further details.

How it works

On receiving the request for an assessment, the co-ordinator allocates two Qualpac assessors and two auditors to the unit or ward. The auditors have agreed that their requirements are a quiet, well-lit room with a desk or other suitable worktop. The notes to be audited are selected by the unit staff and it is essential that they are complete: any charts used to record information pertaining to the nursing care of the individual must be included. Usually the notes are audited retrospectively and therefore the ward needs to be warned in advance to enable the notes to be retrieved from the records office. Staff seem to expect that the notes of the patients under observation by the Qualpac assessors will be the sets required for audit.

The audit usually takes place at the same time as the Qualpac assessment although this is not essential. The time taken to complete the audit is about two and a half hours. Ward staff need to be reassured that it is not an inspection imposed by management or the authority and that the service is provided by clinical nurses for their professional colleagues. In order to allay any anxiety the arrangements are made with the Sister well in advance so that any queries can be answered before the assessment takes place. The names of the auditors are given to the ward and they wear mufti for the occasion. The reaction of the nursing teams to the auditors on arrival has on the whole been friendly and co-operative in spite of any lingering anxiety.

The nursing background of the auditors is varied; most are currently working in community hospitals or as district nurses, however this does not affect their ability to audit records of special wards or units within the general field of nursing.

Nursing records are not standardised throughout the District and the first task the auditor faces is to find her way around the nursing notes. Some units use a very simple Kardex system with space for personal details on the front sheet and then space for the nursing record, with no other set formula. There are some Kardex-type records which have headings listing activities of daily living and social details which encourage the taking of a nursing history and making an assessment, of the problems. Records designed to take a history, make an assessment plan and evaluate the care are also in use. It is much easier to examine and measure the standard of care in such notes and generally these have been rated more highly than other types. However, it has also been shown that it is not necessary to have special stationery in order to provide individualised care and some nursing care recorded in the simpler style has achieved a good score as it is the content which is measured rather than the format.

A variety of different charts are in use and auditors have to ensure in each ward that they have been given the complete set. On one occasion there appeared to be a gap in the information contained with the notes and on enquiry it was discovered that in order to reduce the bulk, charts used in the early stages had been removed. In these circumstances auditors have to use their judgement as to the scoring.

In view of the increased demand for the service and limited numbers of auditors, a certain amount of discussion has taken place regarding the necessity or desirability of allocating two auditors to each assessment. On balance, however, it was agreed that there were certain advantages in having two auditors. Obviously, it halves the time taken to complete the task but it also enables the auditors to consult each other when doubts arise, especially when handwriting proves difficult to read. In the event of any real concern about the safety of the level of care as portrayed in the notes, there is a second opinion close at hand. Most auditors have found it useful to be able to discuss their findings and provide support for each other.

Reading the notes in order to audit them can be difficult. Some nurses write in such an illegible hand as to cause one to wonder how anyone else could carry out the instructions or continue the care. Variations of handwriting, colour of ink and colour of paper can all prove tiring to the eye but, on the other hand, some handwriting is very easy to read and pleasant to look at. There are nurses whose record-keeping can make the auditors feel that they know the patient while others leave them wondering whether the nurses knew the patient at all. Even in situations where the notes are poorly kept, good entries by just one nurse over a period of days can influence the overall gradings for a set of notes. Abbreviations are used by some people but may mean different things to different people, thereby affecting the scores given. Apparently, some nursing charts are not regarded as a permanent part of the records and are removed or destroyed after the patient's discharge and this will be reflected in the final scores. Fortunately, it is possible to ascertain this type of information from staff at the time of the audit and allowance can be made when writing the report. Care is shared by relatives at times, especially when children are being nursed, and there is sometimes a question whether this has been fully recorded. Patients who are readmitted frequently to the same ward for treatment appear to be so familiar that an initial assessment is not always evident, thus presenting difficulty in deciding whether appropriate care has been given. Those units which have a relatively short length of stay fare less well in the section relating to discharge plans, although one can understand the difficulties in this setting. Although audit is usually carried out retrospectively, there are wards and units where this is difficult, for instance, in places such as coronary care or recovery units, as patients are transferred to other wards rather than discharged; in such circumstances current records are used for the audit. Such wards gain a certain advantage as items which are not appropriate are graded as if they were dealt with and score top marks; this system is to ensure that scores are not adversely affected in wards where certain procedures are not carried out.

The benefits of audit

Interesting trends have been identified in the audits undertaken to date, certain types of wards or units achieving better scores in specific functions. Function 1, the execution of doctor's legal orders, is usually found to be good. In the acute surgical and medical wards the section relating to observation of signs and symptoms tends to score much higher marks than the sections relating to the psychological care of the patient and to advice and teaching. This probably seems to be entirely predictable but, unless measured objectively, the ward staff are unlikely to be aware of the true picture.

Nursing audit also enables the individual primary nurse to look at her own practice. On one or two occasions it has been quite clear that certain nurses have special skills and qualities, especially in writing care plans. If these are identified, the potential for educating the rest of the team is enormous. A recent audit has highlighted this particular situation and the ward sister has been able to motivate the particular nurse towards teaching the junior members of the team. Another nurse, through her notes, demonstrated that she is quite possessive about her patients and has been able to recognise that she needs to involve the family more. Specialist wards have sometimes devised a standard care plan, especially in respect of pre and postoperative care, and this at least ensures that all aspects are identified and planned for and that care is not left to the mercy of staff without the necessary background knowledge. Audit will reveal whether these plans are being sensitively used and that adaptations to suit individual needs are made. It would be all too easy to become complacent because standard care plans were in use.

The report on the audit is formally written in confidence to the person who requested the audit, with the recommendation that the findings are shared with the rest of the team. An agreement was reached during the training sessions that no information would be given to line managers, in order to prevent the abuse of the audit by using it as a form of discipline. The reports are all in the same format, beginning with a description of the audit team and its training and the Phaneuf method of auditing records. Each section is described separately with examples of excellent care or unsafe care being cited, and the grading for the section.

An overall grading for the sets of notes is given with a table and graph illustrating the variations. Comments about any factors which may have adversely affected the outcome are made, together with an offer to audit further notes, return at a later date or discuss the report if the nurse requesting the audit feels that there were mitigating circumstances which prevented an accurate picture being obtained. Response to the report has been interesting, one report which was thought to be below average apparently provoked no reaction from the staff, another average report resulted in the reply 'well of course we do a lot more but we do not write it down'.

The effects of feedback to the nursing teams is still to be measured in most cases but there are several indicators to its value. The standard of record-keeping improves in content even where the format remains unchanged. Nursing care concentrates on the individual. The report serves to reinforce the better aspects of care and encourage greater awareness of those areas that have been neglected. The need for the nurse to be a co-ordinator, planner, supervisor and teacher is shown to be essential to good nursing practice and thus supports her in her professional role. Accountability towards patient, profession and public is more likely to be achieved when the documentation shows the reason for each action, the expected outcome and the evaluation of the care: nursing audit highlights these points.

The reasons given by those requesting an assessment including an audit are varied. Some have been requested by newly-appointed ward sisters who wish to have a measurement of the quality of care which was delivered when they took up their posts, in order to compare with any progress they might make. Sisters who have been promoted to senior sister with responsibility for a group of wards have requested an audit for their unit with a view to identifying the strengths and weaknesses within it. Sisters appointed with a specific responsibility for clinical practice and development wish to monitor the success of their educational programmes in terms of improved standards. Nursing audit can also improve morale among nursing teams because examples of excellent and good nursing care are mentioned in the report.

The use of audit within nursing teams has much to recommend it. Nurses are expected to maintain and improve standards of care; those best qualified to judge standards are fellow professionals and the record of care delivered is one way of doing so. Accountability for one's actions is one mark of the profession and nursing audit allows for this. Resources remain as scarce as ever and need to be used most effectively and audit can show whether efforts are directed in the most appropriate way. One example was that of a young woman about to be discharged who displayed symptoms indicating that no improvement was taking place and that she was not following initial advice. In spite of this no extra examination took place, no further advice or counselling was given and 48 hours after discharge she was readmitted for further treatment. Attention to pre-discharge education might well improve the outcome in this unit. Evaluation of changes in ward management, models of care, and reporting mechanisms can be achieved by the use of audit. All nurses from time to time need to have an indication that their practice remains as good as possible and audit can motivate and support them. One ward audited in the early stages of the programme has requested a repeat audit in order to measure progress.

Audit can be used to measure the care given by district nurses. An extension of this might be a Primary Nurse in a ward or unit who requests individual assessment for her personal use. As a forerunner to undertaking a course, or further training, it would provide a baseline against which any changes could be measured.

Auditors themselves have obtained positive benefits from being involved in the assessments. Their own record keeping improves and they have the opportunity to look objectively at other systems of note storage and care planning. All professional nurses feel a sense of achievement when they feel that they have been instrumental in improving standards of care, whether it is on the ward they have examined or because of the impact of their own practice.

The continued request for assessment is an indication of the value of the assessment to the ward teams and equally encouraging is the recent interest shown by those who wish to train as auditors. In the initial stages it appeared that nursing audit did not have the same appeal as the Qualpac observation but experience is proving that audit has much to offer both to those audited and to the auditors. Most important, however, is the potential for ensuring that nursing care is regularly reviewed. This is particularly important in the light of changes resulting from reorganisation of the health services and likely changes in nurse education.

Nurses are exhorted to become more conscious of research and to implement findings when appropriate. Changes in practice need to be monitored and evaluated and Phaneuf's audit may enable this to be effected more easily.

References

Hegyvary S T & Haussman R K D (1976) Monitoring nursing care quality. *Journal of Nursing Administration*, **6**(9)

Jelinek D Haussman R & Hegyvary S (1974) *A Methodology for Monitoring Quality of Nursing Care*. Bethesda: U.S. Department of Education, Health & Welfare

Lelean S (1973) *Ready for Report Nurse?* London: Royal College of Nursing

Lesnik M J & Anderson B E (1955) *Nursing Practice and the Laboratory*. Philadelphia: Lippincott

Marrinner A (1979) *The Nursing Process*. St. Louis: C.V. Mosby

Mayers M Norby R B & Watson A B (1977) *Quality Assurance for Patient Care—Nursing Perspectives* . New York: Appleton-Century-Crofts

Phaneuf M (1976) *The Nursing Audit*. New York: Appleton-Century-Crofts

5
Monitor

LEONARD A GOLDSTONE

We frequently hear pronouncements such as 'standards of nursing care are falling' or 'British nursing is the best in the world'. How do we know? Those who make statements of this kind presumably are looking at some clear indicators of the quality of care. Are these indicators comprehensive, valid and reliable? Further enquiry usually reveals that the statements have been made out of a conviction or personal belief rather than being founded on systematic examination of the facts. Sometimes we are told that 'the quality of nursing care cannot be measured'. Worryingly, it is often the same people who have informed us that standards are falling or that British nursing is best who provide these incompatible statements.

Those who make judgements on the quality of nursing must rely on some implicit criteria. Can we elicit these, expand them, increase their objectivity and comprehensiveness? Those who say that quality cannot be measured may well agree that there are some identifiable aspects of quality whose presence or absence can be observed objectively, and which can act as a pointer to a more general view of quality. Monitor seeks to make explicit criteria which are implicit in the quality statements of many nurses, and relies on aspects of nursing that are observable as having occurred (or not). *Monitor – an Index of the Quality of Nursing Care for Acute Medical and Surgical Wards* is based on research which has demonstrated that there are aspects of nursing care which can be easily and objectively observed, and which are valid and reliable indicators of quality. The methodology is applied to the care of individual patients, and so by using if for all the patients on a ward (or a certain random sample) an index of the quality of care on a ward is available. The quality within a health authority may be estimated too.

The 'Patient Monitor' assesses the quality of nursing in relation to four areas of care:

53

1   planning and assessment;
2   physical care;
3   non-physical care; and
4   evaluation of care.

A further index, contained within Monitor, assesses the quality of practice, procedure and management of the ward: this 'Ward-Monitor' is independent of the 'Patient-Monitor'.

The complete system, collectively titled Monitor, is available in a single publication, presented as a book. Health authorities use it without external help or consultation; even the calculations are done simply – a computer is not necessary.

The background to Monitor

Monitor is an adaptation for the UK of the Rush Medicus Nursing Process Methodology. The first step of the extensive research was an in-depth examination of a large number of studies and instruments concerned with measuring the quality of nursing care. From an initial list of approximately 900 quality-related items of nursing care, a final set of 257 evaluation criteria was developed by the Rush Medicus researchers. Pilot-testing on 8 patient units in two hospitals for five months, and further development in 107 patient units distributed over 19 hospitals for six months, was completed.

Monitor was subsequently researched in the UK in 32 acute medical and surgical wards within the North Western Regional Health Authority. Although it was developed against a scenario of the nursing process, it has been successfully used in wards where task allocation is the mode of operation.

In the USA, the Rush Medicus instrument is one of the most widely-tested and most thoroughly-analysed methodologies for indicating the quality of nursing care.

The structure of Monitor

Monitor contains four separate patient-based questionnaires, each one related to a different category of patient dependency, ie. Group I relates to patients requiring minimal nursing care, Group II to patients requiring average nursing care, Group III to patients requiring above-average nursing care, and Group IV relates to patients requiring maximum nursing care. Monitor also contains a questionnaire for the 'ward'.

Each questionnaire contains questions demanding simple observation to which the response is usually 'yes' or 'no'. Monitor consists of checklists relating to the presence or absence of quality-related observable phenomena. Not all questions can be answered with a full, unqualified 'yes'. Accordingly, there are several alternative versions, eg. 'yes, incomplete', 'yes, sometimes', 'yes, partially'. We have scored such responses as half a mark compared with one mark for a full 'yes'. The scoring system focuses on the applicable questions, and the percentage of those to which a 'yes' response is obtained. The closer to 100 per cent the better the care being delivered.

Nurses who have used Monitor agree that it is comprehensive and valid. Our tests have shown that the questions and responses are framed so that any two 'assessors' using the checklists will obtain very close agreement, and very similar scores. The assessors are senior, clinically experienced nurses, but they do not assess in those areas which are their direct responsibility.

Since its introduction Monitor has been widely used in the UK and has demonstrated clear inequalities in the scores obtained in different health authorities, ranging from a typical score of 47 per cent in the lowest scoring health authority to 82 per cent in the highest, with even greater variation for individual wards and patients. Monitor does not embrace all aspects and dimensions of quality in nursing care. It focuses on 'process' rather than structure or outcome. Nevertheless, within the confines of its coverage it provides valuable information for nurses and demonstrates inequality and the need for training and education.

Content of Monitor

The items in Monitor are based on a master list of over 200 criteria. These are split into four sub-lists, each appropriate to patients of different dependency levels. Thus there are 81 items for Category I patients (minimal care), 107 items for Category II (average care), 149 items for Category III (above average care) and 118 items for Category IV (maximum or intensive care). In addition, there is a list of 43 quality related items for the ward as a whole – the 'ward Monitor'. Monitor for patients follows the structure of the nursing process, although this does not need to be operating to use Monitor.

The criteria for assessing quality hinge on the extent to which nurses realise and use their comprehensive roles to meet patients' needs. Of course the process of nursing is a continuum of 'caring', but a useful starting point is an examination of the assessment of the patient's needs and problems, upon which the plan of care is based. The care should refer to whatever physical needs the patient has, for example, hygiene, mobility, treatments, diet, fluids, bowel care and others. The non-physical needs are equally important and typically encompass 'information', 'education', emotional support, privacy, and so on. Monitor checks that all the appropriate care, from the stage of assessment and planning through to implementation and evaluation has been completed. The major sections of Monitor are:

(a)   Planning nursing care.
(b)   Meeting the patient's physical needs.
(c)   Meeting the patient's non-physical needs (includes psychological, emotional, social needs).
(d)   Evaluation of the nursing care.

Each major section includes a series of pertinent questions. These are described in Table 5.1. For each of the subheadings there are between three and seven specific questions in Monitor.

Table 5.1   Subjects covered in Monitor

Section A   Planning and Assessment

Assessing the patient on admission
Information collected on admission
Assessment of patient's current condition
Co-ordination of nursing care with medical care plan

Section B   Physical Care

Protecting the patient from accident and injury
Provision of physical comfort and rest
Needs for hygiene
Needs for nutrition and fluid balance
Needs for elimination

Section C   Non-Physical Care

Orientation to hospital facilities on admission
Nursing staff courtesy
Patient's privacy and civil rights
Consideration to patient's emotional and psychological wellbeing
Measures of health maintenance and ill-prevention are taught
Involvement of patient's family and/or carers

Section D   Evaluation of Care

Appropriateness and evaluation of objectives
Patient's response to treatment is evaluated

The number of questions under each section is not constant.
   Table 5.2 demonstrates how the numbers vary according to the dependency of the patient. There are around 25 questions on planning care for each group, but the physical care questions vary from 16 for Category I patients up to 74 for Category III, and the non-physical care questions from 17 for Category IV to 35 for Category III. Evaluation is usually dealt with in approximately 15 questions as shown in Table 5.2

Table 5.2   The number of Monitor questions per section for the four categories of patients

Number of questions in Monitor	Category of patient			
	I	*II*	*III*	*IV*
A Planning Care	23	24	28	25
B Physical Needs	16	34	74	65
C Non-Physical Needs	28	34	35	17
D Evaluating Care	13	15	15	14

The development of Monitor

The original Rush Medicus methodology was intensively tested for validity and reliability in the USA, and our own work confirms its acceptability. It was first carefully 'anglicised' and then scrutinised by over 100 active nurses in the acute medical and surgical areas, and then systematically tested within the North-Western Region. Initial trials of Monitor in the North-Western Region were based on whether the questions generated for use in the US were applicable to the NHS. Preliminary discussions with ward sisters and charge nurses in local hospitals helped to remove reference to procedures inapplicable to UK nursing.

The first Monitor trials were conducted in two surgical and three medical wards. The wards were quite ordinary – they had between two and four consultants, around 25 beds and were using task allocation. Medical students and student nurses were present in all wards, but pupil nurses were present only in three. Ward clerks and domestic assistants were available in all wards, and physiotherapy services were provided both on and off the ward in most cases. Occupational therapy was a regular service only in three wards. A CSSD service was available in all five wards. In three wards 'plated meals' were provided while the other two had 'trayed meals'. There was only one case where the meals were not exclusively served by the nurses. The ward design in four of the wards was typically Nightingale-style but the fifth, Ward E, consisted of six open bays. Monitor was applied to a sample of patients on each of the five wards. Three patients, in each of the four dependency categories were randomly selected.

The results from the five wards, in relation to the four patient categories, are presented in Table 5.3, which shows the mean percentage of 'yes' responses obtained for the patients on each ward.

Table 5.3   Monitor results from initial trial on five wards

	Wards				
	A	B	C	D	E
Category I	80.9	–	68.0	59.2	50.4
Category II	81.2	74.3	66.3	55.8	54.4
Category III	82.5	72.1	67.4	62.5	38.9
Category IV	–	66.0	65.3	58.2	42.0
Ward Mean	81.6	72.5	66.4	60.0	48.5

The uniformity of figures within each ward is striking, except for Ward E, which is the lowest scoring ward. The range, from 81.6 per cent down to 48.5 per cent indicates an enormous variation in the quality of nursing care provided and one which has been repeated in subsequent studies. These trials showed that no major revisions to the Rush Medicus questions were needed, but considerable attention to language was required.

The test on the five wards, while interesting, was conducted to discover the relevance and applicability of the Monitor questions. It was also felt important to check the reliability of the results from one assessor to another. It is important that results obained by assessor A can be reproduced by assessor B.

A sample of four wards in two teaching hospitals was chosen for the reliability trial. On each of these wards observers A and B – both qualified and experienced nurses – carried out the full Monitor evaluation on the same patients. The results are shown in Table 5.4, and indicate a remarkable level of agreement.

Table 5.4   The similarity of the results from two assessors using Monitor on 4 wards – represented as percentages

Mean % Agreement Question by Question	Hospital X		Hospital Y	
	Ward XL	Ward XM	Ward YN	Ward YP
Category I	93.8%	91.7%	98.4%	93.8%
Category II	96.8%	99.1%	95.6%	98.2%
Category III	95.4%	–	95.8%	91.1%
Category IV	95.5%	95.6%	92.6%	–

The reliability study also entailed the two assessors independently using the ward Monitor questionnaire: the results are presented in Table 5.5.

Table 5.5   The similarity of the results from two assessors using the ward-Monitor questionnaire on 4 wards

	Hospital X		Hospital Y	
	Ward XL	Ward XM	Ward YN	Ward YP
% Agreement, Question by Question	97.5	80	97.5	97.5

The lower figure, (80 per cent), on Ward XM is explained by the fact that the observers were not present at exactly the same time, due to different speeds at which the patient Monitors were filled in. Even so, by the standards of most research instruments, 80 per cent agreement is still very high.

When we examine in detail the scores obtained for each patient, we find a remarkable similarity. The mean difference between the assessors is 1.1 per cent, with 71.4 per cent of the differences recorded being under 3 per cent, and 82.9 per cent being less than 5 per cent. There is only one difference recorded over 8.5 per cent and this was in a ward where standards of care were seriously amiss.

Overall, taking together the minimal recorded difference in scores, the high percentage of agreement question by question and the high correlation between the assessors, we felt sufficiently confident to apply Monitor more widely.

A sample of 10 per cent (approximately) of acute medical and surgical wards in the North West region, were chosen on the basis of their willingness to try

Table 5.6   North Western region nurse staffing levels system: information matrix (pilot study)

Ward	% of Direct Care	Nursing Activity per 24 hours: Minutes of Direct Care per Dependency Category				Monitor Scores		% Score Nurse Satisfaction	Ward Type and Beds
		I	II	III	IV	Ward	Patients		
1	50	71	107	206	206	48	53	77	FS 19
2	47	54	92	104	270	51	49	X	M 35
3	69	47	108	174	315	65	61	61	FS 29
4	74	53	95	207	313	67	60	X	FM 28
5	61	51	92	194	311	87	72	70	FM 27
6	40	45	77	203	—	69	78	X	MM 31
7	51	37	141	170	418	66	61	X	FM 30
8	50	75	135	218	218	68	73	59	FM 24
9	56	29	99	165	267	66	72	54	FS 22
10	55	29	58	171	316	76	66	72	MM 28
11	57	37	74	130	215	79	73	78	FS 27
12	46	52	99	177	276	88	65	57	FS 32
13	53	85	102	204	544	80	82	71	FS 26
14	54	86	138	267	430	76	60	X	MS 22
All Wards Mean Score	54.5	53.6	1.9	3.5	5.9	70.4	66.1	—	– 27

out Monitor; scores were obtained for each of the wards using a random sample of approximately three patients per category in each ward. Table 5.6 shows the Monitor scores, together with some other management information collected. The nurse satisfaction score is a percentage obtained from a simple questionnaire in which the nurses were asked to rate their own satisfaction with the care they were able to provide.

Perhaps the most interesting feature of Table 5.6 is the lack of correlation between the columns! The only two columns with any degree of association are Monitor for the ward, and Monitor for the patients, between which, as might be expected, is a simple correlation of 0.62. Wards 1 and 2 both devote more minutes to Category I patients than average, but considerably less to the more ill patients in Categories III and IV, and a lesser percentage of nursing time in general to direct care, resulting in a very low level of service as measured by both Monitors. Ward 13 in contrast with the highest Monitor score for patients and a similarly high score for the ward, also devotes the highest minutes of direct care to its patients, especially those most ill. There are some interesting contrasts: in Wards 5 and 12 a very high score for the ward – suggesting a well organised, tidy ward – is not matched by a high patient score. It appears that the ward receives a lot of attention, but the patients' needs are not always met.

Finally, it is noticeable that the range of scores, ie. from 49 per cent to 82 per cent is the same as that obtained in the five pilot wards, confirming Monitor's ability to discriminate. In all of the work up to this point a mean Monitor score of 66 per cent emerged. This was reported in the final preparatory study of nine wards in District X. Moreover, there was considerable consistency within the results from District X. They ranged from 59 per cent to 71 per cent but most were in the 60s. The results from District X were very 'average' and are described more fully below.

The good, the bad and the average

The variations in the Monitor index found between wards in the development work has been mirrored closely by that found between health authorities. Monitor is the first tool which makes comparisons feasible. Table 5.7 shows the average Monitor score for patients and for wards in three health authorities in the UK. A sample of wards in each health authority was studied: there were usually 4 patients in each of the four patient categories per ward.

Table 5.7   Average Monitor scores for Health Authorities

	Mean Monitor Score (Patients)	Mean Monitor Score (Wards)
Authority W	47	63
Authority Y	66	81
Authority X	82	89

Authority Y represents the most common picture – a score for patients averaging 66 per cent – the same average as that obtained in all previous work.

The range, from 47 per cent to 82 per cent, is typical of the 'worst' – 'best' wards, formerly observed.

Table 5.8 presents the results for each ward, within the Health Authorities W, X and Y. Evidently, there is considerable variation, around the mean scores for the worst Health Authority (W), less variation around the mean in Health Authority X, and least in Health Authority Y. Perhaps the most striking feature of the table is that patients in a medical ward in Authority W score on average 38 per cent on Monitor, whilst their counterparts in Authority X on Ward L score 87 per cent on average. Put another way, for every 100 questions about care to which a 'yes' response was obtained, Ward L exceeds Ward A by 49 'yes' responses. Another interesting feature of the table is that the 'best' ward in Authority W scores approximately the same as the worst ward in Authority Y, and, moving along this continuum of scores, the best ward in Y scores approximately the same as the 'worst' ward in Authority X. Despite this wide variation in standards it should be repeated that the most common pattern of scores is that found in Authority Y, and this indicates a considerable potential for 'better' nursing in many health authorities.

Table 5.8   Mean Monitor score for patients on each ward

Authority W Wards		Authority Y Wards		Authority X Wards	
A	38	R	69	L	87
B	41	S	67	M	84
C	42	T	64	N	83
S	44	U	59	P	82
E	55	V	66	Q	70
F	60	W	70	Mean	82
Mean	47	X	71		
		Y	59		
		Z	65		
		Mean	66		

It is possible to be much more specific in reporting back from a Monitor study. Table 5.9 shows the level of detail suitable for use by a unit manager or nursing officer for a particular ward, in this case Ward F. Table 5.9 presents the Monitor score for each aspect of care for each category of patient, plus the average score for the dependency groups (bottom row) and the aspects of care (last column on right) independently. Finally the overall score for the ward (ie. 60 per cent) is presented. The managers would probably need to read the information in this table in reverse order, starting at the bottom right hand corner.

The overall score of 60 per cent is achieved by the averaging of low scores 41 per cent on planning and 51 per cent on evaluation, with high scores on physical care (76 per cent) and non-physical care (72 per cent). However, even the high score 76 per cent is unevenly distributed over the patients, being averaged from 90 per cent for Category I patients, 81 per cent and 84 per cent for the middle categories, and only 65 per cent for Category IV. It therefore appears that the most dependent patients obtain the lowest physical care score, and the least dependent obtain the highest – indicating the need for serious review, and change for the nursing of the most ill patients. The low planning score is very erratic too.

Table 5.9   Monitor results for ward F

| Ward F | Category of Patient | | | | |
Aspect of Care	I	II	III	IV	All Patients
A Planning	26	48	29	54	41
B Physical	90	81	84	65	76
C Non-physical	61	83	83	63	72
D Evaluation	59	47	63	46	51
Overall Care	53	66	61	58	60

A 'prescription' for the ward could include detailed attention to the use of records, and planning of care as a means of individualizing care to most patients' needs; attention to the physical and non-physical needs of the most ill patients in Category IV and to the non-physical needs of Category I patients. Obviously, the non-physical needs of these extreme-dependency groups are quite different, and the factors involved must be made explicit. Part of this process involves the nursing officer and ward sister in perusing the actual Monitor document in detail (question by question/patient by patient) and developing a strategy for improvement.

Attention to the evaluation of care is also required. The timescale for improvements will vary. It is important to set realistic and objective goals and in this way the managers can demonstrate and impel the principles of the process of nursing.

Table 5.10 shows the results obtained for Ward P, in which there were no Category I patients.

Table 5.10   Monitor results for ward P

| | Category of Patient | | | | |
Aspect of Care	I	II	III	IV	All Patients
A Planning	–	76	77	85	77
B Physical	–	86	85	100	88
C Non-physical	–	83	81	93	83
D Evaluation	–	75	82	83	77
Overall Care	–	81	82	93	82

The overall score of 82 per cent is made up of scores of over 80 per cent for Categories II and III patients, and 93 per cent for Category IV patients. The latter are the most dependent, for whom the physical care score is 100 per cent.

Compare this with Ward A results (Table 5.11).

Table 5.11   Monitor results for ward A

| | Category of Patient | | | | |
	I	II	III	IV	All Patients
A Planning	22	33	14	23	25
B Physical	38	60	59	30	56
C Non-physical	30	53	54	27	41
D Evaluation	41	44	35	42	42
Overall Care	31	52	43	29	38

Alarmingly, Ward A scored only 29 per cent for its Category IV patients overall, and 30 per cent for the physical care. We have found that despite academic discussion on what Monitor actually 'measures', and what it excludes, the differences observed can be so dramatic that enormous improvement can be clearly signposted.

The reality of using Monitor is that change can be demonstrated to be required, and the nature of the change clearly indicated. Many health authorities using Monitor have produced either a catalogue of undeniable improvements in care resulting from Monitor, and/or a single fundamental change for which Monitor was the catalyst.

Steps prior to using Monitor

1   Monitor requires assessment of the work of nurses and puts some questions to patients. Health authorities wishing to utilise Monitor are recommended to consider consultation in advance with the appropriate trades unions, and with the Ethical Committee.

2   A steering group of ward sisters and nursing officers should be set up under strongly-committed chairmanship at a very early stage to study the content of Monitor in detail. It is usually best if the steering group includes the 'assessors' who will actually fill in the Monitor documents. The assessors (two per ward) should be experienced and senior nurses who are not line managers of the wards being studied, and who will be acceptable to the ward sisters or charge nurses.

3   A seminar should be conducted to explain to ward staff who will be involved the reasons for using Monitor, its structure, nature and practical details. We have found it helpful to make copies of Monitor available at this seminar, and to permit ward staff to take the copies back to the wards for further perusal. Whilst this can result in some 'window dressing' to create an improved picture to present to the Monitor assessors, the reduction in anxiety among ward staff because of the familiarity obtained is usually preferable to keeping the questions in Monitor as a secret.

Any improvements to patient care obtained simply by leaving a copy of Monitor for staff to peruse can only be of benefit. Additionally copies of the *Guide to Monitor* should be made freely available.

4   The steering group and assessors will need approximately five meetings, each of up to two hours' duration, to go through Monitor in depth, question by question. The object is to ascertain that there is uniformity of understanding of the questions. The Category III Monitor questions should be used for this exercise as they are the longest batch of questions and will show up any problems in understanding or interpretation. The meetings should be fortnightly to permit thought, discussion and some actual practice of using Monitor on a few patients to take place between the meetings. The role of the group leader is crucial. He or she must overcome the minor details which present difficulty and facilitate agreement and common understanding of 'difficult' questions. The many health authorities which use Monitor usually find up to ten questions which take considerable discussion, needing strong chairmanship.

The ten questions will not be the same in each district. It is almost always possible to resolve difficulties during the five meetings, and progress is considerably quicker in the later meetings. If absolutely necessary, minor changes to questions and omission of irrelevant or inappropriate questions should be agreed on. No major revisions or additions should be considered because Monitor has had extensive testing for validity and reliability in its present form, and completely new questions would not be as well researched. They would also render results not directly comparable with those from other user health authorities.

The Steering Group therefore should agree on a minimum-change-basis the form of Monitor to be used. All copies will need editing, to be identical, using a bold, felt-tipped pen. The overriding criteria for editing must be to allow for specific local policy or conditions.

5   The question of who the assessors should be has been dealt with in several ways. In large health authorities staff from similar wards in other hospitals have moved across to the study ward. Nursing officers and ward sisters with recent or current relevant experience find the exercise of being a Monitor assessor to be valuable educational experience. It is usually best to use at least two assessors per ward, and thus at least one should be very familiar with the speciality. In small health authorities we have observed the use of staff from other wards in the same hospital, but sometimes this presents problems where a small nursing community is involved. And we have also seen successful collaboration between several neighbouring authorities who together run the whole Monitor exercise and train a 'pool' of roving assessors who can go to any ward in any of the districts. In this way training costs are spread and the necessary skills can usually be found.

6   The acute medical and surgical wards chosen for study should receive notice of the planned approximate dates of the study, which should be set

bearing in mind planned staff holidays and student/pupil nurse allocation. The ward at the time of the study should be operating as normally or typically as possible. Thus the ward sister or charge nurse should be asked on the actual study day to agree that workload level, patient mix and staffing provision are not untypical.

The assessors should not proceed if the ward sister or charge nurse is uneasy about the particular circumstances of the day. Since Monitor involves putting some questions to patients, the Steering Group should agree a method of informing patients about Monitor.

Steps in using Monitor

1   Having obtained the assent of ward staff to proceed the assessors should, in close co-operation with the ward sister/charge nurse agree the dependency classification of each patient on the ward, and complete the patient classification list. Each patient is placed into one of four categories, and then the particular set of appropriate questions can be selected and put. For some patients, such as those in a relatively stable condition, the dependency classification may be agreed on the day prior to the study day.

2   All the patients on the ward should be included in the study. This is possible over approximately two days for two assessors in a 25 bed ward. Alternatively, a sample of approximately three patients in each dependency group should be selected at random, without reference to the ward sister/charge nurse, and without reference to the patient's records. No judgements on the suitability for inclusion of certain patients are permitted – the decision should be impersonal and mechanical. In the case of the small number of patients who are likely to be classified as Dependency IV it may be necessary to include all of them, and there may still be less than three.

Patients' initials (or a code, such as the last four digits of the patients' hospital number) should then be entered onto the appropriate Monitor sheets.

3   Each assessor should then answer the questions for the groups he/she has chosen. One Monitor document should suffice for all the patients in any one dependency grouping. It is likely that the division of work will be:

Assessor A: Dependencies I, III
Assessor B: Dependency II, the likely largest group, and
               Dependency IV, the smallest group

4   The Monitor questions for the ward/unit should be put by the assessor who completes the patient-based Monitor first.

Scoring Monitor

Each patient-based Monitor has four sections, A, B, C and D. Each of these can be scored separately for each patient, and an overall score for the patient can also be obtained. The majority of Monitor questions have three main responses: 'no', 'yes', 'not applicable/not available'. In a small number of cases the 'yes' response is differentiated further such as: 'yes, always', 'yes, complete', etc., all of which count as a full 'yes'. Additionally there is a 'lesser' version, such as: 'yes, sometimes', 'yes, in part, 'yes, incomplete, etc., all of which count as half a 'yes'.

We therefore score as follows:

'Yes', 'yes, always', 'yes, complete', etc.	1
'Yes, sometimes', 'yes, incomplete', etc.	½
'No'	0

Responses such as 'not applicable/not available' should be marked X in the 'score' box. To obtain the per cent index for each section A, B, C and D, and for all the care of the patient the following steps are performed:

1   deduct number of inapplicable responses from the total number of questions to obtain the number of applicable responses;
2   obtain the total score by adding up all the 'yes' responses (1 point each) and the 'yes, incomplete' type of responses (½ point each);
3   divide the total score by the number of applicable responses, and multiply by 100 to produce a percentage, which is the required index.

The INDEX produced, whether for a particular section or overall, represents the percentage of 'yes' responses achieved, and is thus an index of quality achievement.

Scoring System for the Ward

Either

In a ward with up to 25 beds it is feasible to include all patients in the study. The score for the ward is the mean of all the patient scores. This is obtained by adding up the individual patient scores and dividing this total by the number of patients on the ward.

It should be expected that about three days' of work by two assessors will be required to conduct Monitor on the ward.

Or

In wards with more than 25 beds, or on smaller wards where assessor time is limited, a sample of patients will suffice.

It has been suggested earlier that three patients in each dependency classification be chosen completely at random, without reference to the ward sister, and in a completely mechanical way. In the case of Category IV patients the study may have to accept less than three patients, because such patients are likely to be in a separate intensive care unit.

The scoring should be done as follows: for each dependency group obtain the mean of the scores of the patients in that group—this provides four group means. Suppose, for example, that these are:

Category	I	II	III	IV
Mean	70	72	74.6	69.2

Now check how many patients are currently on the ward in each category (ie. *all* patients in ward, including those used in the sample): suppose these are as follows:

Category	I	II	III	IV
Number of patients	4	12	5	2

We then treat the four patients in Category I as each having scored 70, and thus achieved 4 × 70 = 280 points between them. The 12 patients in Category II are treated as though each scored 72, making 12 × 72 = 864 points, and so on.

The total estimated score on the ward is thus

$$
\begin{array}{rl}
 & 4 \times 70 \\
+ & 12 \times 72 \\
+ & 5 \times 74.6 \\
+ & 2 \times 69.2 \\
\hline
= & 1655.4 \\
\hline
\end{array}
$$

This total score of 1655.4 is divided by the total number of patients (4 + 12 + 5 + 2 = 23) to produce the overall score of $\frac{1655.4}{23} = 71.79$

The score recorded for the patients on this ward is then rounded to 72.

In exactly the same way as the overall score is calculated, we can also work out the overall ward score for a specific section, such as Section A (Planning Nursing Care).

The following steps can then be taken:

1   Completed questionnaires and scores for individual patients should be discussed in detail with the ward sister and relevant nursing officers by the assessors. Attention to 'no' responses can be given and a plan for remedial action (if necessary) can be drawn up.

2   After a suitable period – minimum six months – allowing for changes in the light of the discussions on the completed questionnaires, the study may be remounted. It is recommended that under normal circumstances Monitor should be applied approximately once per year.

The consequences of Monitor

Monitor has been widely used in the UK and abroad since its publication in 1984, and many positive and appreciative communications have been made to the authors by users. In several cases, extensive teaching programmes have been started as a result of the Monitor exercise; the nursing process has been both introduced and re-introduced; patient information has noticeably improved and patient care has undoubtedly benefited because nurses widely report adopting practices which Monitor included but for which they had scored 'no'; nurses frequently report improved confidence in their work after being 'Monitored'; and the concept and practice of practical quality assurance seem to have arrived through the medium of Monitor. We believe Monitor to be only the first step, and because it has been taken successfully, many health authorities now routinely use Monitor and have moved on to explore other new tools.

We mentioned earlier that the only abilities required to score Monitor were the abilities to count and calculate percentages. Most recently a computer programme has become available which does this too – leaving the scorers only the job in inputting the data. The microcomputer then prints out all scores for patients, groups and wards automatically, as shown in Table 5.12.

Table 5.12   North West nurse staffing levels project

	Monitor scores Category 1 patients				
	Patient				*AV*
	1022	*1024*	*1025*	*1026*	
A Planning	65.2	39.1	43.4	56.5	51.0
B Physical	62.5	62.5	68.7	62.5	64.0
C Non-physical	65.5	68.9	65.5	65.5	66.3
D Evaluation	61.5	69.2	69.2	61.5	65.3
Overall	64.2	59.2	60.4	61.7	61.3

New developments recently completed are a version of Monitor for use in geriatric wards, and a cousin Monitor for use in district nursing. Versions for psychiatric wards and paediatric wards will be available in 1987, and the research for midwifery and health visiting versions is in progress at Leeds Polytechnic for planned publication in 1989.

A recent article in the *Nursing Times* perhaps indicates best the current position on Monitor: 'Monitor is proving popular with ward sisters and nurses because it shows exactly where care is failing and where improvements should be focussed. It is popular with managers because it indicates which wards may be failing and why.'

References

Ball J A Goldstone L A & Collier M M (1984) *Criteria for Care: The Manual of the North West Nurse Staffing Levels Project.* Newcastle-upon-Tyne Products Ltd

Goldstone L A Ball J A & Collier M M (1983) *Monitor: An Index of the Quality of Nursing Care for Acute Medical and Surgical Wards.* Newcastle-upon-Tyne Polytechnic Products Ltd

Illsley V A & Goldstone L A (1986) *Guide to Monitor.* Newcastle upon Tyne Polytechnic Products Ltd

Jelinek R C Haussman R K D Hegyvary S T & Newman J F (1974) *A Methodology for Monitoring Quality of Nursing care.* DHEW Pub No (HRA), 76–25

Jelinek R C Haussman R K D Hegyvary S T & Newman J F (1976) *Monitoring Quality of Nursing Care. Part 2: Assessment and Study of Correlates.* DHEW Pub No (HRA), 76–7

Jelinek R C Haussman R K D & Hegyvary S T (1977) *Monitoring Quality of Nursing Care. Part 3: Professional Review for Nursing – An Empirical Investigation.* DHEW Pub No (HRA), 77–70

Slack W P (1985) Standards of care. *Nursing Times,* 29 May, 28–32

6

Outcome Measures

ALAN PEARSON

Outcome measures are aimed at eliciting what the 'end result' of nursing is, and to judge whether or not this is satisfactory. For example, if a patient is admitted with a pressure sore two inches in diameter and discharged with the sore totally healed after 10 days, the assumption will be that care is satisfactory. Such measures have to be related to stated standards, which are often difficult to establish. In the case of the pressure sore the appropriate length of time in which healing should take place would have to be determined. If it takes 10 months, does this indicate poor quality care, or is the fact that healing eventually occurred sufficient to indicate that care was satisfactory. Similarly, if the sore does not heal at all in a debilitated, weak and thin individual, does this indicate poor care? Whilst desired outcomes of care can often be set, every receiver of nursing care is an individual and thus a whole range of unique factors surround each one. Mayers (1978) suggests that outcome evaluation can best be applied by comparing the specific goals set in individual care plans with the final outcome of care. The patients' feelings of satisfaction with care are also a measure of outcome.

Measuring and judging the outcomes of nursing care is an attractive method of determining quality, and there is a growing desire in some quarters for nursing to concentrate on this area of evaluation. Because of its complexity, however, little appears in the literature on how to do this. The three methods which may be feasible are:

— setting outcome standards for specific patient groups and comparing outcome with the stated standards;
— comparing stated goals on individualised care plans with the eventual outcome;
— post-care patient interviews/questionnaires.

71

Setting outcome criteria

This involves 'sorting' patients' problems into specific groups, and then determining what outcomes should arise if care is to be seen to be successful. Usually, groups are determined by medical diagnosis, procedures carried out, or specific problems which commonly occur.

Medical diagnosis

For example, experts in diabetes may agree that a newly-diagnosed diabetic who requires daily insulin injections, and who is otherwise physically fit, and reasonably intelligent, should be able accurately to:

— test his own blood glucose levels and interpret the result;
— describe diabetes and explain its effect on the body;
— state the daily dietary schedule to be followed;
— draw up and give his own insulin injection;

within 7–10 days. If he is able to do this within the time scale, and he does not become hypo or hyperglycaemic, the assumption would be that nursing care was effective.

Procedure carried out

For example, it may be agreed that the otherwise healthy person who undergoes an abdominal hysterectomy will be discharged in five or six days, and on discharge will:

1   demonstrate self-examination of the breasts;
2   manage to give own medication and know each drug and its action;
3   state time for follow up appointment with gynaecologist;
4   state what she anticipates will happen six weeks after discharge;
5   the family will describe provision for return to home situation;
6   have a clean dry incision line.

Similarly, the well-prepared pre-operative patient may be expected to:

— sleep for 5–7 hours, uninterrupted, with sedation, during the night prior to surgery;
— demonstrate coughing and deep breathing exercises prior to surgery; and so on.

Specific problems

Desired outcomes for specific problems may be set. In the example of the pressure sore cited earlier, a healed sore within four weeks may be seen as a reasonable outcome, or a rate of healing no less than a reduction of 1 cm in the diameter of the sore each week may be set as an acceptable standard.

Although setting generally-agreed outcomes for groups of people is extremely difficult to do, it is possible for individual teams, units, or hospitals to work on such a programme and develop outcome protocols. There is a growing political desire for this to occur, and recent claims by politicians and health service leaders that health care is more efficient than in the past are often based on outcome evaluations. For example, the fact that more patients are discharged home after successful joint replacement operations is seen as a measure of increased quality.

There is, however, a major flaw in using outcome evaluation as a single indicator of quality – very often a successful outcome may arise *in spite* of the care given, rather than because of it. Furthermore, many patients will not be able to achieve outcome criteria within the time schedule set, but staff may exert pressure on them to do so in order to be seen to be effective. Those who fail to reach the desired outcomes may well do so because of other factors, and poor quality may be presumed when in fact nursing care has been of a high standard.

This approach to outcome evaluation, although it has a general usefulness in many cases, is perhaps too simple to evaluate the complexity of nursing intervention. It assumes a stance which denies individual differences and sometimes dehumanises the human service of nursing.

Comparing individualised goals with eventual outcome

Mayers (1978) argues that outcome evaluation is best carried out in nursing by concentrating on the desired outcome determined for each individual patient. Because of the huge differences in people, blanket criteria for every person admitted to a hospital with a specific problem is seen to be inappropriate to nursing. In this approach, emphasis is placed on the use of problem-solving in nursing practice, which includes continuing evaluation. Using the nursing process, the patient and nurse work together to arrive at an individualised assessment and identification of problems. Using this assessment, appropriate desired outcomes are stated for each problem and care is prescribed. The eventual outcome of care can therefore be identified and compared with the desired outcome. For example, the care plan in Figure 6.1 clearly lists the problems of Mrs Stevens. The desired, reasonable outcomes are also stated.

When the patient is discharged the initial problem statement can be compared with the desired outcome statement, and a judgement made on whether or not the eventual outcome indicates that care was satisfactory. In the case of the first problem, if Mrs Stevens' pain level on the painometer was 9 on discharge, the nursing intervention could be judged to be poor; if it was 1, to be very good; and if it was 4 or 5, to be satisfactory.

Outcome evaluation using this method is time-consuming, and is dependent upon the correct application of the nursing process. It demands that both problem statements and desired outcomes are stated in observable (if possible, measurable) terms, and that the outcomes are realistic. Few clinical nurses are able to plan care in this way at present and frequently desired outcomes are vague, based on unsubstantiated evidence, and orientated towards the goals of the nurse, rather than to the desired outcome in the patient's condition, ability, or behaviour.

Fig 6.1

Care Plan		
Name: Mrs P Stevens	*Primary Nurse:* Tony Brown	
Problem	*Desired outcome*	*Nursing Action*
1 Pain in hips and knees (level 7 on painometer on assessment)	Pain level on use of painometer will be constant at 5 or less for 24 hours	
2 Cannot walk well unaided – walked from bed to dayroom with help of two nurses. Unable to walk back to bed.	Will be able to walk from bed to ward entrance and back with walking frame, without assistance of nurse.	
3 Unable to sleep for more than 2 hours without waking.	Will sleep for at least 6 hours without waking for three successive nights.	

Like all outcome measures, it again assumes that the outcome arose because of the care and this cannot always be assumed. Nevertheless, Mayers' method is a useful tool as part of a quality assurance programme, and it allows for individual differences in patients.

Patient interviews/questionnaires

Many nurses argue that the receiver of nursing care is perhaps the best person to evaluate its quality. On first sight, this appears logical, but Hall (1966) argues that patients are likely to accept what is given with gratitude because of their vulnerability, and that they often have little experience of different standards of care and are thus unable to make comparisons. Patients also have expectations of nursing which may not reflect high quality. For example, in one small study by Pearson (1985), being woken at 6am and nurses being 'too busy to talk to me' were seen as acceptable because patients expected nurses to be busy, and saw routine as a sign of efficiency.

Seeking the opinion of patients does have a role, however, in evaluating the nursing care received, and the satisfaction of the consumer is one outcome which is desirable. Rosso (1984) argues that seeking the '*beliefs* of patients about the care they have received' is an effective outcome measure. She notes that patients are more likely to respond openly after discharge rather than during their stay in hospital through fear that sanctions may be imposed against them if they say 'bad' things about nurses.

To elicit patient satisfaction levels accurately, the interview or questionnaire should use specific questions about specific areas of care, and the patient should understand the purpose of the questions – that is, to assess quality and attempt to improve it. Hall *et al* (1975) used a closed-question approach to seek information about the quality of direct patient services, which included the physical environment, attitudes of nurses, and speed in which requests for assistance were met.

Conclusion

Reliable and tested outcome measures in nursing are not yet fully developed, although it is likely that there will be increased pressure on nurses to evaluate the outcomes of their care. Although it is logical to say that the major aim of health care is to achieve a successful outcome – whether that be satisfied patient, a healed wound, a reduction in pain, or a change in the patient's behaviour – and that outcomes are essential criteria for measuring quality, outcome alone is too superficial and simplistic a measure by which to judge the quality of nursing.

References

Hall L E (1966) Another view of nursing care and quality. In Straub M & Parker K (eds) *Continuity of Patient Care: the Nurses Role*, 47–61. Washington DC: Catholic University of America Press

Hall L E Alfano G J Rifkin E & Levine H S (1975) *Longitudinal Effects of an Experimental Nursing Process*. New York: Loeb Center for Nursing

Mayers M (1978) *A Systematic Approach to the Nursing Care Plan*. New York: Appleton-Century-Crofts

Pearson A (1985) *The Effects of Introducing New Norms in a Nursing Unit and an Analysis of the Process of Change*. Unpublished Ph D Thesis, University of London: Golsmiths College, Department of Social Science and Administration

Rosso M F (1984) Knowledge of practice: the state of clinical research. In Willis, L.D. & Linwood, M.E. (eds) *Measuring the Quality of Care*, 43–65. Edinburgh: Churchill Livingstone

7
The Role of Innovation in Raising the Quality of Nursing

ALAN PEARSON

The essential rider in quality assurance is *changing poor practice into good practice*. Measuring and judging in itself is of little use if the service to the patient or client remains unchanged. Changing things – or innovation – is essential both as the final step in the quality assurance process, and in the wider sense of introducing useful change. Change in itself is always a problem to many human beings, and nurses are no exception. High quality or high standards are usually synonomous with a team or organisation which is innovative and open to change. Discussions in the literature frequently ignore this crucial ingredient of promoting high quality care – the fostering of innovation.

Innovation and quality

The 'quality' of nursing is, as has already been said, an especially difficult phenomenon to define, describe, and measure because it is a human service which *must* always hang on to an element of subjectivity and intuition. There are aspects of 'good' nursing which are almost intangible and maddeningly subtle. This creates huge difficulties in an age where quantification, certainty, and proof are seen as essential. In *The Little Prince*, Antoine de Saint-Exupery shows this clearly in the story:

> 'Grown-ups love figures. When you tell them that you have made a new friend they never ask you any questions about essential matters. They never say to you, what does his voice sound like? What games does he love best? Does he collect butterflies? Instead they demand: How old is he? How many brothers has he? How much does he weigh? How much money does his father make? Only from these figures do they think they have learnt anything about him'.

The friend's voice, his favourite games, his interest in butterflies are about quality. Without this subjective, almost woolly dimension, it is impossible to know anything about this writer's friend. So it is with nursing, an activity all about people. Safety, effective wound healing, discharge home quickly, and such like may all contribute towards indicating quality but the less measurable, less objective side to the story is vital to establish what true quality care is.

Quite recently, I was planning to leave home with my family at midnight. I intended to drive down overnight to catch a boat the following morning to reach a holiday destination. In the evening, at about 9.30, my brother rang to say that my mother had been admitted to hospital. He assured me that all was well and said that of course I should still go on holiday. I rang the hospital to find out more. It was by then 10 o'clock at night and I had worked in that hospital before and I could imagine how the staff would be quite busy and how they wouldn't really welcome a telephone call. So when I was put through to the ward I apologised for such a late enquiry. The staff nurse, however, was very helpful, very kind, gave me lots of information and suggested quite strongly that I should speak to my mother on the portable telephone before going on holiday. I left on holiday the next day and in the evening of the next day, my mother died in the hospital. It really was a lot of comfort to me to know that I had at least spoken to her for about half an hour before she died, because I hadn't seen her for a few months.

Now this is the sort of thing that reflects quality. It cannot be counted or measured but nor can it be discounted as being simply icing on the cake or frivolous luxury. It is a mark of high quality.

Innovation in clinical nursing, not directly related to the result of quality measurement, currently focus on this human, subjective side of practice, and fostering innovation which promotes a greater development of the less tangible and measurable area of the nurturing role of the nurse are just as important in assuring quality as well-ordered measurement and judgement.

Innovation

Innovation, says the dictionary, is 'Making changes; introducing new practices'. An expanded definition is making changes or introducing new practices in a creative way and with success. But innovation is simply changing and all nurses innovate all of the time to a greater or to a lesser degree. An 'innovative person' is generally somebody who is more open than usual to change and when nurses talk about an innovation they refer to something that is positive and related to being go-ahead, dynamic and creative and which ultimately leads to an improvement.

It is clear that innovation is an absolute necessity in promoting quality. Introducing a quality assurance programme is, in itself, an innovation. Trying to use Monitor or Qualpacs or some form of audit or outcome measure in a ward or community setting is, in itself, an innovation. In the search for quality, one seeks to find out how things are and to change them to make them better: that, in itself, is an innovation. Innovation in nursing is either the generation and trying out of new ideas or the creation and introduction of new methods that will bring into reality some of the ideas that are currently valued in nursing.

Most nurses are aware of the new ideology being promoted in nursing as a result of changes in the society they live in. Because nursing is a human service and social change is an ever-present process, nurses have to innovate all the time. They have been exhorted to change at least since Florence Nightingale came on the scene and no doubt it will always be so. Currently, there is enormous evidence that the direct care-giving nurse needs to re-think things and adopt a number of radical changes if the recipients of her care are to be given something which they really want, need and have a right to.

The observations by sociologists such as Davies (1976; 1977) and Menzies (1960), Stein (1978), Stannard (1973) and many, many more, the findings of studies on nursing such as those by Towell & Stockwell (1972) and the feedback from patient surveys such as those carried out by the Royal Commission in 1978, by Cartwright in 1964 and by Raphael in 1969 all suggest that nursing needs to change for the sake of the patients. The nursing discovered by such studies was not marked by its high quality. The current drive is for nurses who give care to adopt a holistic care-orientated model and to be less reliant on a medical cure-orientated model which will emphasise:

1   the individual and his needs rather than routinisation;
2   the accountability of the nurse to the patient;
3   practice which is knowledge-based;
4   the development of a close relationship centred on partnership between nurse and patient;
5   the use of a systematic problem-solving or need-meeting process.

Nursing leaders believe these ideas are of vital importance and official bodies such as the National Boards and The World Health Organisation assert that nurses must try to adopt these new values of practice norms to reflect them. The whole intention is to achieve quality care (although based on a professional philosophical stance).

Adopting practice norms to reflect these new values is the function of innovation. Because of the human side of nursing, there actually is no set check-list that a nurse can work through in order to demonstrate that she has adopted these values. The door is open for many, many varied styles of nursing that would all adequately deliver care that meets these ideas. Real innovation involves clinical nurses looking at the ideas, being creative and translating them into practice in various ways that will suit the particular client group.

Changes can be brought about by the insistence of supervisors that clinical staff should carry them out; for example, the introduction of a problem-solving or needs-meeting process. This has happened in various places up and down the country in a most unsatisfactory way when lists of questions have been compiled, typed and called 'the nursing process forms'. These forms have then been issued to clinical nurses who have been told 'Fill them in and you will be doing the nursing process'. Such a procedure cannot really be regarded as an innovation because it is not necessarily successful and has not been seen to be a positive contribution to quality.

Three basic change strategies have been described by Chin & Benne (1976):

(a)   The rational empirical approach assumes that people are likely to view innovation positively and work towards it if they are given the basic facts and empirical information and if this evidence 'indicates that they will derive some benefit from the innovation'. This strategy therefore requires a logical argument and its supporting evidence to those to be involved.
(b)   The normative re-educative approach believes that 'people have values, norms and attitudes that influence, if not direct, their behaviour' (Archer et al 1984). Given the arguments, and facts to support them, is therefore seen to be not enough to persuade people to change and the normative re-educative line focuses on 'helping people to re-examine their values in the hope that they will come to view situations differently'.
(c)   Finally, the power-coercive approach is applying power vested in individuals who are superior within the institution. This latter approach is the one followed in the previous example of the introduction of the nursing process. Real, lasting innovation virtually always takes place through the normative re-educative approach in clinical settings. It involves actually talking to clinical nurses, allowing them to express their feelings, allowing them to accept or reject current ideology, encouraging them to be creative in applying those ideas that they can identify with and it inevitably, according to Archer et al leads to a change not only in practice but in the whole climate of work. Any individual, – a nurse, a policeman, a patient, or whoever – actually begins to grow when he feels that he can contribute to the working of the team.

The general feeling in nursing is that the ideas mentioned above could lead to the sort of quality that nurses would wish to have. But ideas alone are of little use. They cannot be forced upon people and telling them about it will not lead to a change of practice and therefore a change in quality of care.

The change in quality, the change in the reality of practice, is what happens through innovation. More importantly, innovation in practice is something that will always be needed, as knowledge develops and community needs change. It can only be achieved by qualified nurses who have the power and ability to innovate.

A climate for change or innovation

How does one get innovation under way in a clincial unit? The run-down geriatric hospital down the road that is understaffed, has highly-dependent patients and poor facilities – how does one get innovation into a place like that? Or into an acute ward of 30 beds with patients who stay for three days, and with 10 on the theatre list every day – how can one get innovation in there? I think that there are a few pointers to what can be done.

Firstly, innovation takes place with staff who are capable of being innovators and this requires people with a broad education who can see beyond the fulfilment of tasks. So the first point is that we really need educated nurses.

Pembrey suggests that quality care depends on two things – qualified practitioners and the quality of the professional education in both the initial preparation and in the continuing mastery of the discipline throughout professional life.

Secondly, innovation never takes place in an environment where power-coercion is the norm and rule-books are wielded over staff. The philosophy of the organisation must value the contribution of clinical nurses and their individual accountability to clients. If clinical nurses, and therefore the potential innovators, feel that they function within a climate where they are worth something and where they will be given permission to initiate change, then innovation is more likely to occur.

Lastly, I would suggest that really good innovators tend to be the mavericks of nursing. So, an innovative unit often depends on managers employing those who do not always toe the line, who sometimes dissent, who do want to challenge and who do want to innovate.

In her analysis of reality shock, Kramer (1974) suggests that four types of nurse emerge out of such shock. Firstly, there are the lateral arabesques – that is those who, when they are faced with the reality of practice, move out sideways; they tend to hop from job to job or they move away from clinical practice into other fields such as teaching or research. The second group she calls the rutters: that is, those who face the reality of practice and who take on board the norms that they face, who are professionally inactive and who strive to maintain the status quo.

The third group are the organisation men and women. They are ones who are both professionally committed and career-orientated. They are very loyal to the organisation but are keen on innovation, tend to climb the ladder fairly quickly and achieve fairly senior positions. Kramer's fourth group are the bi-cultural troublemakers – those who hold in their heads the ideals and identify with them but also identify with the organisation and tend to question frequently. These people are valued both by their supervisors and by the organisation and worried by it. It seems that, according to Archer et al, Kramer's third and fourth groups are those who are the innovators. So the third pointer is actively to recruit organisation-men and women and bi-cultural troublemakers. We need more troublemakers in nursing.

To conclude, I suggest that innovation is actually the most important activity that contributes towards quality in direct care. A creative unit with people in it who innovate is one in which quality can be achieved. Evaluating the structure and outcome of nursing and feeding this back to clinical staff is, of course, essential for quality, but developing the actual process of nursing through innovation and from the feedback from such quality estimations is absolutely crucial to quality care. Nursing needs a creative environment in which to function if it is to achieve full quality.

Schweer (1972) purports that 'if we truly seek to keep creativity alive, we must continue to nourish the conditions in which creativity flourishes' and describes four aspects of the creative process; and it is these that we have to promote in order to allow innovation to take place. She says that we need to infiltrate the environment for nursing with:

1   an emphasis on openness to new ideas;
2   a focus or direction on the achievement of quality;
3   a discipline within individuals of themselves to be creative; and
4   a feeling that permission is given for the creative products to be institutionalised if they are found to be effective.

References

Archer S E Kelly C D & Bisch S A (1984) *Implementing Change in Communities – A Collaborative Process.* St Louis: C V Mosby

Berg H (1974) Nursing audit and outcome criteria. *Nursing Clinics of North America,* **9**(2)

Bloch D (1975) Evaluation of nursing care in terms of process and outcome. *Nursing Research,* **24**(4)

Cartwright A (1964) *Human Relations and Hospital Care.* London: Routledge & Kegan Paul

Chin R & Benne K D (1976) General strategies for effecting changes. In Bennis W Benne K & Chin R (eds) *The Planning of Change.* New York: Rhinehart & Winston

Davies C (1976) Experience of dependency and control in work: the case of nurses. *Journal of Advanced Nursing,* **1**(4), 273–282

Davies C (1977) Continuities in the development of hospital nursing in Britain. *Journal of Advanced Nursing,* **1**(5), 479–493

Doughty D B & Mash N J (1977) *Nursing Audit.* Philadelphia: Davis

Egleston E M (1980) New JCAH standard on quality assurance. *Nursing Research,* **29**(2), 113–114

Hall L E (1966) Another view of nursing care and quality. In Straub M & Parker K (eds) *Continuity of Patient Care: the Role of Nurses,* pp 47–61. Washington, D.C: Catholic University of America Press

Hegyvary S T & Haussman R K D (1976) Monitoring nursing care quality. *Journal of Nursing Administration,* **6**(9), 11.3–9

Hover J & Zimmer M J (1978) Nursing quality assurance: the Wisconsin system. *Nursing Outlook,* **26**(4), 242–248

Jelinek D Haussman R & Hegyvary S (1974) *A Methodology for Monitoring Quality of Nursing Care.* Bethesda: U.S. Department of Health, Education & Welfare

Kings English Dictionary (1930) London: British Book Company

Kramer M (1974) *Reality Shock: Why nurses leave Nursing.* St Louis: C V Mosby

Mayers M Norby R B & Watson A B (1977) *Quality Assurance for Patient Care – Nursing Perspectives.* New York: Appleton-Century-Crofts

Menzies I E P (1960) Nurses under stress: a social system functioning as a defence against anxiety. *International Nursing Review,* **7**(6), 9–16

Raphael W (1969) *Patients and their Hospitals.* London: Kings Fund

Royal College of Nursing (1981) *Towards Standards.* London: R C N

Royal Commission on the National Health Service – Report (1979) London: H M S O

Schmadl J C (1979) Quality assurance: examination of the concept. *Nursing Outlook,* **27**(7), 462–465

Schweer J E (1972) *Creative Teaching in Clinical Nursing.* St Louis: C V Mosby

Stannard C (1973) Old folks and dirty work: the social conditions for patient abuse in a nursing home. *Social Problems,* **20**, 329–342.

Stein L (1978) The doctor-nurse game. In Dingwall R & McIntosh J (eds) *Readings in the Sociology of Nursing.* pp 107–117. Edinburgh: Churchill Livingstone

Towell & Stockwell F (1972) *The Unpopular Patient.* London: R C N

8

The Way Forward

ALAN PEARSON

In the preceding chapters we have tried to explain what is meant by standard-setting and quality assurance, and have presented the view that quality assurance in nursing should be a form of peer review. The specific methods of Qualpacs, Nursing Audit, Monitor and outcome measures have been described, as has the role of innovation in assuring quality. This final chapter presents a practical illustration of combining a number of methods to create a quality assurance programme based on the notion of peer review in nursing.

The way forward

With the increased pressure on health service agencies to institute quality assurance (or control) there is a very real possibility, if clinical nurses continue to distance themselves from involvement in them, that peer review and the opportunity for nurses really to improve services to patients will be lost, and that nursing practice will be monitored and regulated by non-nurses or nurses divorced from the reality of direct patient care. Thus, the only way forward is for clinical nurses to take current methods on board and use them in an appropriate way as a form of peer review. In addition, the need to foster innovation and reject the notion that nursing should be standardised and controlled will have to be strongly voiced.

How this will be done in different areas and units has to be determined by the practitioners who work in them, and their colleagues in management and education. As an example of how this can begin, it is useful to present an outline of the early attempts at introducing quality assurance as a form of peer review in nursing carried out in one health district (Oxfordshire) in the United Kingdom.

Early development

Although this programme is in its early stages of development, it focuses clearly on the clinical nurse's accountability for the quality of care she/he gives, and on quality assurance as peer review. Froede & Bain (1976) suggest the following schema for setting up a quality assurance programme (Figure 8.1).

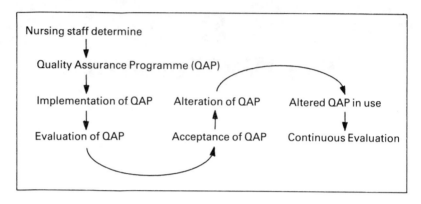

Fig. 8.1

This shows how a programme undergoes continuous development as a result of evaluation. The Oxfordshire programme will undoubtedly change as it is continuously evaluated, but it demonstrates how clinical nurses, working as peer review groups, can engage in quality assurance.

A trial quality assurance programme was begun in 1984. It looked at concurrent process evaluation by direct observation of care and retrospective process evaluation, through audit of the nursing records. The combination of the two was chosen to give an overall picture of quality of care and in what areas improvement could be made. Qualpacs and Phaneuf's Nursing Audit were the tools used.

Assessors and auditors

An initial group of practising clinical nurses were trained; an auditing induction and training package of four half-days and extended practical work was conducted and 11 nurses completed a two-day Qualpacs assessors course and a period of extended practical work. A large part of the training involved actual assessments by the whole group, which demanded agreement on acceptable standards. An offshoot of Audit/Qualpac training was the growing awareness amongst the nurses involved of a shortfall in quality in their own practice, and subsequent efforts to change this.

Following this trial, a pilot programme centred on a quality assurance team was developed to include all units which wished to participate, and a clinical nurse specialist was co-opted as a trainer and to act as overall programme co-ordinator. A pilot service was then offered to clinical nurses which would provide them with an assessment by their peers of the quality of their care, in order to promote change.

The team consisted of a self-regulating group of Qualpac assessors and nursing auditors, with a leader elected by the group from amongst their number. Requests for assessment, which could be single or a continuing series, were accepted from clinical nurses, ie. sisters and senior sisters/nursing officers. The assessment reports were sent to the nurse(s) who requested it, and a copy was held by the co-ordinator.

As the programme existed to support and help clinical nurses, reports were only passed to nurse managers by the clinical nurse who requested the assessment, but if serious deficiencies in care were discovered, the assessors/auditors had the right to insist that the requesting nurse discussed the report with nurse management.

The pilot programme gained a great deal of acceptance from clinical nurses, and generated an interest in quality and serious attempts to change poor practice. It was, however, limited in its effectiveness because it did not include any structural or outcome evaluation, and it was still largely an ad hoc, informal activity without full organisational support.

Setting up the formal programme

A steering group was convened by the District Nursing Officer to evaluate the current quality assurance pilot programme and to recommend any modifications with a view to setting up a formal strategy to assess quality of nursing. The outcome of these discussions was the amalgamation of a number of tools to be used as a framework for peer review.

Principles

(a) It was felt that quality *assurance* was much more than quality *measurement* or *monitoring*. The latter two merely report what is happening, whereas quality assurance aims to change practice which is seen to be poor. Therefore, the approach whereby clinical nurses request an assessment by other clinical nurses was seen as crucial in assuring quality. The findings are seen as credible and they are fed back to clinical staff without fear of punitive action by management. Furthermore, the report is fed back to the whole ward team, and this creates an impetus for change.

(b) Qualpacs and nursing audit are valid and reliable tools to measure process but there is a need to incorporate structure and outcome measures.

(c) If it is seen that quality assurance can be used to promote better nursing care, then a planned programme should be adopted by all units.

Tools to be used in the programme

Structure

The Monitor audit assessment tool has a section titled 'ward-centred questions' which, with some modification, gives a useful framework for a structure evaluation which has been tested for reliability and validity.

Process

Qualpacs and Phaneuf's Audit are useful measures of process. Qualpacs is concurrent and Audit retrospective, and the combination of both is a useful framework to use which has been tested for reliability and validity.

Outcome

Outcome measures are not as yet well developed. The Patient Service Checklist, tested in the USA and used in the Burford study (Pearson 1985), has some limited usefulness. However, it was felt that funds should be sought from the locally-organised research scheme to mount a study to develop outcome measures. Thus, at present, a quality measurement package which combines parts of Monitor, Qualpacs, Audit and Patient Service Checklist was adopted to be used in the quality assurance programme. At a later date, further outcome measures will be incorporated into the tool.

The complete assessment package will be found at the end of this chapter.

Proposed organisation of the programme

Each unit is asked to 'twin' with another, as follows: Unit 1 with Unit 2, Unit 3 with Unit 4, and so on, and the assessment of each unit is carried out by clinical nurses from its 'twin' unit. Not only is this organisationally easier but it also increases the awareness by clinical nurses of activities in other units.

Requests for assessments from senior clinical nurses are made to the co-ordinator, who directs appropriate assessors, and receives the final report. The report is then sent to the requestor who is *required* to share it with the clinical team and *advised* to share it with nurse management.

Provision is made for one assessment per year for every ward and department in Oxfordshire. The programme does not, at this stage, include a provision for district nursing, health visiting, family planning or occupational health.

Conclusion

High-quality nursing care is the right of all patients, and is the responsibility of all nurses who give it. Clinical nurses can either reject this responsibility, and therefore allow others to regulate nursing practice, or they can accept it with enthusiasm and strive for quality in a realistic way, rather than ignore the current drive to set standards and measure quality in the hope that it will go away. The quality of nursing care depends on the quality and creativity of the nurses who give it. Quality is excellence in care and, as Brodt (1970) comments: 'the choice between excellence or obsolescence provides the answer to enquiries regarding the future role of the nurse'.

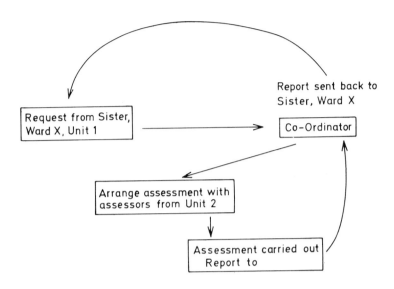

References

Brodt DE (1970) Excellence or obsolescence: the choice for nursing. *Nursing Forum*, **9**, 19–26

Froede D J & Bain R J (1976) *Quality Assurance Programmes and Controls in Nursing*. St Louis: C V Mosby

Pearson A (1985) *The Effects of Introducing New Norms in a Nursing Unit and an Analysis of the Process of Change*. Unpublished Ph D thesis, University of London: Goldsmiths' College, Department of Social Science and Administration

QUALITY ASSURANCE PACKAGE
(Wards & Departments)
Oxfordshire Health Authority

Contents

ASSESSMENT FRONT SHEET

1 Name of Ward/Department _____

2 Person requesting assessment and
  to whom report should be sent _____

  _____

  _____

3 Average daily bed occupancy
  (for Outpatient Departments, average daily attendance) _____

4 Average patient length of stay _____

5 Total staffing establishment (in WTE)

  Sisters _____

  RGNs _____

  Nursing Auxiliaries _____

  Orderlies _____

  Domestics _____

  Clerical Officers _____

  Others (specify) _____

PART I WARD/DEPARTMENT PROFILE

(To be completed by the ward sister/charge nurse in consultation with the assessors)

1 Main speciality on ward _____

2 Sex   Male ☐   Female ☐   Mixed ☐

3 Bed complement _____

4 Are extra beds put on the ward?   Often ☐   Sometimes ☐   Never ☐

5 How many extra beds? _____

6 (Surgical Units)
   Number of operating sessions per week _____

   Operation days _____

   Average number of operations per week _____

7 How many consultants have beds on the ward?

   Name _____   Number of beds _____

   _____   _____

   _____   _____

   _____   _____

   _____   _____

8 When do consultants' rounds take place, and how long do they last?

Consultant	Day(s)	Time	Duration
_____	_____	_____	_____
_____	_____	_____	_____
_____	_____	_____	_____
_____	_____	_____	_____
_____	_____	_____	_____
_____	_____	_____	_____
_____	_____	_____	_____

9   Is the ward used for teaching?

    Medical Students   Yes ☐   No ☐

    Student Nurses   Yes ☐   No ☐

    Pupil Nurses   Yes ☐   No ☐

10   Hours Worked: how many nursing staff are normally allocated to the ward (excluding learners)?

	Full Time	Part Time (give weekly hours)
Sisters/Charge Nurses		
Staff Nurses		
Senior SENs		
Nursing Auxiliaries		

11   Do you have use of a nurse bank   Yes ☐   No ☐

12   Are bank nurses used on a regular basis on your ward? If yes, please give details such as particular shifts, particular days bank nurses are used.

    Yes ☐   No ☐

13   Is any basic training given to nursing auxiliaries?   Yes ☐   No ☐

14   How are nursing tasks assigned?

    Team Nursing ☐   Patient Allocation ☐   Task allocation ☐

    Primary Nursing ☐   Combination of above, please explain ☐

15   Do you have the services of a ward clerk?   Yes ☐   No ☐

16   What hours does the ward clerk work?   _____

17   Is the ward clerk shared with another ward?   Yes ☐   No ☐

18   Is the ward clerk paid from the nursing budget?   Yes ☐   No ☐

19   What hours do the domestic assistants work?   _____

20   Is there any relief for sickness/absence/
    holidays of ward clerks?   Yes ☐   No ☐

21   Is there any relief for sickness/absence/
    holidays of domestic assistants?   Yes ☐   No ☐

22   Is the portering service satisfactory?   Yes ☐   No ☐

    If not, in what way? _____

23   Are physiotherapy services satisfactory?   Yes ☐   No ☐

    If not, in what way? _____

24   Are occupational therapy services satisfactory?   Yes ☐   No ☐

     If not, in what way? _____

25   Is a Central Sterile Supply Service satisfactory?   Yes ☐   No ☐

     If not, in what way? _____

26   Is the provision of food satisfactory?   Yes ☐   No ☐

     If not, in what way? _____

27   Who *usually* serves the meals?   Nurses ☐   Other staff ☐   Both ☐

28   Are nurses regularly involved in the collection of the following items?

	Yes	No		Yes	No	
Blood from blood bank			Linen			
Drugs			Specimens			
Stores			Other, please state			

29   Are there any restrictions on patients' meal-times, which in turn affect the organisation of nursing tasks?   Yes ☐   No ☐

     If yes, please explain _____

30   What are the visiting hours? _____

31   Are outpatients seen on the ward?   Usually ☐   Sometimes ☐   Never ☐

32   How many in the past four weeks? _____

33   Is this typical? (If not, please explain)   Yes ☐   No ☐

     _____

34   Are day cases admitted to the ward?   Usually ☐   Sometimes ☐   Never☐

35   How many in the past four weeks? _____

36   Is this typical? (If not, please explain)   Yes ☐   No ☐

     _____

37   Does the ward take emergency admissions?
     Usually ☐   Sometimes ☐   Never ☐

38   What system is used for allocating emergencies to the ward? _____

39   Do nursing staff from the ward escort patients to/from theatre or other units?   Yes ☐   No ☐

40   Do nursing staff from the ward wait with patients in the recovery area?   Usually ☐   Rarely ☐   Never ☐

41   Are there any factors not alluded to above, which you feel have a significant impact on nursing workload? Please state.

_____

42   What do you feel are the three most important factors, on your ward, which limit the amount of time nurses can spend on direct patient care?

1   _____

2   _____

3   _____

PART II   STRUCTURAL REVIEW

Source of information

A   GENERAL

Observe Environment	1	Are oxygen precaution signs posted in readily observed places?	1	No	Yes
				Not applicable	
				SCORE	

Observe Nurse	2	Are wheels locked when patients are helped into and out of wheelchairs?	2	No	Yes
				Not applicable/ Not available	
				SCORE	

Observe Nurse	3	Are wheels locked when patients are helped into or out of bed?	3	No	Yes
				Not applicable/ Not available	
				SCORE	

Observe Nurse	4	When nursing staff discuss patients do they ensure they cannot be overheard by patients or visitors?	4	No	
				Yes, sometimes	
				Yes, always	
				Not available	
				SCORE	

SECTION A				Total questions	
				Total not applicable Q's	
				Total applicable questions	
				Total SCORE	

B   ADMINISTRATIVE & MANAGERIAL PROCEDURES ARE ORGANISED TO HELP THE DELIVERY OF NURSING CARE

1 Nursing reporting follows prescribed standards

Records	(a)	Are nursing notes written about patients as required by hospital policy?	5	No	Yes
				SCORE	
Records	(b)	Are all nursing notes legible?	6	No	Yes
				SCORE	
Records	(c)	Are nursing notes properly signed as required by hospital policy?	7	No	
				Yes, usually	
				Yes, always	
				SCORE	
			8	No	Yes
				SCORE	
Records	(d)	If abbreviations are used in nursing records, are they acceptable to hospital policy?	9	No	Yes
				SCORE	
Ask Nurse	(e)	Does every nurse coming on duty receive a report? TO NURSE IN CHARGE: Using this shift as an example, what personnel on the oncoming shift were given a report?	10	No	Yes
				SCORE	

Ask Nurse   (f)   Are oncoming nurses introduced to patients?
TO NURSE IN CHARGE: Do the day nurse and evening nurse in charge make rounds together at the end of the day shift? (Adapt to other shifts. Were you able to make walking rounds together at the beginning of this shift?)

Ask Nurse	(g)	Do nursing staff report to the nurse in charge at the end of the shift? TO NURSE IN CHARGE: Do you get reports from each person working with you at the end of the shift? Using yesterday as an example, did everyone report to you?	11	No	Yes
				Not available	
				SCORE	

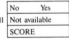

2   Nursing management is provided

Ask Nurse   (a)   Are ward nurses clear about which patients have been assigned to them?

No	Yes
SCORE	

[superscript 12 beside the box]

TO NURSE IN CHARGE: How do you make assignments to nursing staff working with you? If necessary to clarify, ask: Do you tell them which patients are their responsibility in report, or on paper, or by some other means?

Ask Nurse   (b)   Does the nurse in charge allocate patients according to patient needs and capability of nurses?

No	Yes
SCORE	

[superscript 13 beside the box]

TO NURSE: Using today as an example, how did you decide which patients to assign to other members of the nursing staff. Answer 'no' if patients assigned according to numbers of staff. Answer 'yes' if assignment made in consideration of both different levels of staff capabilities and levels of patients needs.

Ask Nurse   (c)   Does the nurse in charge of the ward/unit make rounds on all patients in the unit?

No	Yes
Not available	
SCORE	

[superscript 14 beside the box]

TO NURSE IN CHARGE: During the past 2 days did the nursing officer in charge of the unit make rounds on all patients on the unit?

Ask Nurse   (d)   Are conferences held to plan and co-ordinate the nursing care for specific patients?

No
Yes, less than once a week
Yes, more than once a week
SCORE

[superscript 15 beside the box]

TO NURSE IN CHARGE: Do you hold conferences with staff to plan and co-ordinate nursing care for specific patients? In the past week, how many would you say have been conducted on this unit?
(Patient care conferences refer to any conferences held about a specific patient for the purpose of planning & co-ordinating his care)

Ask Nurse   (e)   Are efforts made to adjust staffing assignments daily according to the severity of the patients' conditions?

No staffing
Yes, or yes patient conditions govern changes
Not applicable
SCORE

[superscript 16 beside the box]

TO NURSE: In the past 2 days have the staff cared for the same patients every day? If yes, tick 'yes' response etc. If no and they have had different assignments, how was the decision made to change assignments? If based on patient's needs, code 'Yes, or yes patients condition governs change'. If not based on severity of patients condition, code 'no'.

3   Clerical services are provided

Records   (a)   Are the records assembled in the correct order?

No	Yes
SCORE	

[superscript 17 beside the box]

Records   (b)   Is there a list of nursing staff on duty for the shift kept at the desk/nursing station?

No	Yes
SCORE	

[superscript 18 beside the box]

Observe Ward Management   (c)   Does a ward clerk (when one is on duty) always answer the ward phone?

No	Yes
Not applicable	
SCORE	

[superscript 19 beside the box]

TO NURSE: In the past 2 days, have clerks on duty always answered the phone at the desk? If nurses have answered the phone code 'no'.

Ask Nurse   (d)   Does a ward clerk (when one is on duty) handle communications with other departments unless direct communication by a nurse is required?

No	Yes
Not applicable	
SCORE	

[superscript 20 beside the box]

TO NURSE: In the past 2 days, when a ward clerk has been on duty has she taken care of all communications with other departments unless direct communication by a nurse is required? Answer 'no' if nurse took care of any routine phone calls or requisitions when clerk on duty.

Records   (e)   Are all routine forms included in the patients' records?
(Check to see that all routine pages are present)

No	Yes
SCORE	

[superscript 21 beside the box]

4 Environmental and support services are provided

			No / Yes SCORE

Observe Environment — (a) Are the patient areas clean? Refers to floor, walls, bedside tables. — 22 | No Yes / SCORE

Observe Environment — (b) Are the toilets clean? — 23 | No Yes / SCORE

Observe Environment — (c) Are the bathrooms clean? — 24 | No Yes / SCORE

Observe Environment — (d) Is rubbish removed from patient areas? — 25 | No Yes / SCORE

Observe Environment — (e) Is all equipment near patient being used or on stand-by basis? — 26 | No Yes / Not applicable / SCORE

Observe Environment — (f) Are electrical devices (apparently) safe *and* disconnected when not in use. (Must be yes to both for 'yes' response) — 27 | No Yes / SCORE

Observe Environment — (g) Is there adequate storage space for equipment? Observe if equipment blocking corridor, taking up excessive space in bathrooms or other non-storage areas. — 28 | No Yes / SCORE

Ask Nurse — (h) Is there an adequate supply of linen provided? TO NURSE: In the past 2 days, have you had enough linen for all your patients? — 29 | No Yes / SCORE

Ask Nurse — (i) Are adequate supplies provided for routine treatments? TO NURSE: In the past 2 days, have you had enough supplies, other than linens for treatments such as dressing changes. — 30 | No Yes / SCORE

Ask Nurse — (j) Does the pharmacy deliver all routine ordered supplies to the ward? TO NURSE: In the past 2 days, have pharmacy personnel delivered all routine and ordered (not emergency) supplies to ward? — 31 | No Yes / SCORE

Ask Nurse — (k) Are supplies from CSSD delivered to the ward? TO NURSE: During the past 2 days have CSSD personnel delivered all supplies to the ward? — 32 | No Yes / SCORE

Observe Environment — (l) Are supplies for handwashing available? — 33 | No Yes / SCORE

SECTION B

Total questions
Total not applicable Q's
Total applicable questions
TOTAL SCORE

C UNIT PROCEDURES ARE FOLLOWED FOR THE PROTECTION OF ALL PATIENTS

34 | No / Yes, always / Not applicable / SCORE

1 Isolation and decontamination procedures are followed

Observe Nurse — (a) Do the nursing staff follow the isolation procedure specified for each isolated patient? If procedure is not *always* followed, code 'no'. — 35 | No / Yes complete / Not applicable / SCORE

Observe Environment — (b) Are measures taken for proper removal of contaminated linen, equipment and waste from isolation rooms? See hospital procedure — 36 | No Yes / Not available/ / Not applicable / SCORE

Observe Nurse — (c) Is the procedure for disposal of dirty/used supplies and equipment followed? (Does not refer to isolation procedure. See hospital procedure) — 37 | No / Yes, sometimes / Not always / Not applicable/ / Not available / SCORE

Ask Nurse   (d)   Are precautions taken by nursing staff to protect patients from known respiratory infections and other communicable diseases?
TO NURSE IN CHARGE: In the past week have you had any incidence of respiratory infections or other communicable diseases on this unit? Are there any measures taken to prevent the spread of infection, such as putting patients in private rooms or requiring staff with respiratory conditions to stay at home?

Observe Nurse   (e)   Do the staff wash their hands between patients?
(If not always done, record 'no')

No	
Yes always	
Not available	38
SCORE	

No	Yes
Not applicable	
SCORE	39

Observe Environment   (f)   Is equipment currently in use clean?

2   The ward is prepared for emergency situations

Ask Nurse   (a)   Are plans for intervention during a cardiac arrest know by the nursing staff? (Applies to medical emergency).

No	
Yes probably	40
Yes definitely	
SCORE	

TO NURSE: What would you do if there were a cardiac arrest on the unit? (Answers include; cleaning airway, cardiopulmonary resuscitation, notifying appropriate personnel, administering medication prescribed in written hospital procedure). If medication is prescribed in written hospital procedure, Score 'Yes definitely' if all four answers given
Score 'Yes probably' if 3 out of 4 answers are given
Score 'No' if 2 or less answers are given

If medication IS NOT prescribed on written hospital procedure;
Score 'Yes definitely' for 3 above answers
Score 'Yes probably' for 2 out of 3 above answers
Score 'No' for 1 or none of above answers

Ask Nurse   (b)   Is the emergency trolley checked in accordance with hospital policy for adequacy of supplies?
TO NURSE: Do you know hospital policy for checking the trolley? If 'no' code 'No'. If yes, when was the trolley checked. Code 'Yes' only if checking done at correct time.

No	
Yes	41
Not available/ Not applicable	
SCORE	

Ask Nurse   (c)   Are actions to be taken in case of fire known by the nursing staff?

No	
Yes probably	42
Yes definitely	
SCORE	

TO NURSE: What would you do if you discover a fire on the ward?
A 'Yes' response *must* include
1   Raise alarm
2   Protect/remove patients
3   Close doors and windows

Code 'Yes' only if all 3 responses are given.

Total questions
Total not applicable Q's
Total applicable questions
TOTAL SCORE

PART III   QUALPACS

QUALITY PATIENT CARE SCALE

INFORMATION FACE SHEET

Patient

Name _____

Record no. _____

Room no. _____ Accommodations _____

Admission date _____

Diagnosis

   Admission _____

         _____

         _____

   Current _____

         _____

         _____

         _____

Condition of patient _____

         _____

         _____

Unit

Name _____ Type _____

Number of Rooms _____

Number of beds _____

Census _____

LEVELS OF CARE (Number of patients in each)

A _____ C _____ E _____

B _____ D _____

PERSONNEL CODE AND CENSUS

Registered Nurse	R_____
Enrolled Nurse	P_____
Nursing Student	SN _____
Pupil Nurse	PN _____
Instructor	I _____
Sister	S_____
Orderly	O _____
Ward Auxiliary	W _____
Aide	A_____
Unknown Initiator	U _____

OTHER PERTINENT DATA:

Date _____

Time of day_____ am/pm

REPORTS: Change of shift _____

          Team_____

          Other _____

Additional notes or questions:

Rater _____

Interactions_____

OUTCOMES: Total item mean score _____

           Total of items used _____

           Score (mean of means) _____

QUALITY PATIENT CARE SCALE

RATER'S NOTES FOR ASSESSMENT AND PLANNING CARE

Patient _____

ORDERS, NEEDS, NURSING ACTIONS

Diet (meals, fluids, nourishment)

Medications

Treatments (dressings, irrigations)

Special care:
(a) colostomy, trach., etc.
(b) skin bath, lotion, etc.
(c) traction, cast
(d) decubiti

Observation of condition
(a) Direct
(b) Monitors (V.S., Pacemakers, etc.)

Diagnostic Tests
(a) On ward
(b) Off ward

Activity (bedrest, ambulation, etc.)

Sensory deficit (blind, aphasic, deaf)

Safety

Teaching patient and family

Socialisation and diversion

Multiple services (referrals, consultations)

Reporting and recording

Planning for continuity of care

Other

QUALITY PATIENT CARE SCALE Qualpacs   Date _____

Patient (name or no.):   Rater (name or no.):
INTERACTIONS RECORD: AM/PM

No.:
Time:

PSYCHOSOCIAL: INDIVIDUAL
Actions directed toward meeting psychosocial needs of individual patients.

	Item number	Best care	Between	Average care	Between	Poorest care	Not applicable	Not observed	Mean score
1 Patient receives nurse's full attention. ★D	1								11-12
2 Patient is given an opportunity to explain his feelings. ★D	2								13-14
3 Patient is approached in a kind, gentle, and friendly manner. ★D	3								15-16
4 Patient's inappropriate behaviour is responded to in a therapeutic manner. ★D	4								17-18
5 Appropriate action is taken in response to anticipated or manifest patient anxiety or distress. ★D/*I	5								19-20
6 Patient receives explanation and verbal reassurance when needed. ★D	6								21-22
7 Patient receives attention from nurse with neither becoming involved in a nontherapeutic way. ★D	7								23-24
8 Patient is given consideration as a member of a family and society. ★D/*I	8								25-26
9 Patient receives attention for his spiritual needs. ★D/*I	9								27-28
10 The rejecting or demanding patient continues to receive acceptance. ★D/*I	10								29-30
11 Patient receives care that communicates worth and dignity of man. ★D	11								31-32
12 The healthy aspects of the patient's personality are utilized. ★D/*I	12								33-34

	Item number	Best care	Between	Average care	Between	Poorest care	Not applicable	Not observed	Mean score
13 An atmosphere of trust, acceptance, and respect is created rather than one of power, prestige, and authority. ★D	13								35-36
14 Appropriate topics for conversation are chosen. ★D	14								37-38
15 The unconscious or nonorientated patient is cared for with the same respectful manner as the conscious patient. ★D	15								39-40

PSYCHOSOCIAL: GROUP
Actions directed toward meeting psychosocial needs of patients as members of a group.

	Item number	Best care	Between	Average care	Between	Poorest care	Not applicable	Not observed	Mean score
AREA 1 MEAN									41-42-43
16 Patient as a member of a group receives warmth, interest and attention from the staff. ★D	16								44-45
17 Patient receives the help necessary to accept limits of his behaviour that are essential to group welfare. ★D	17								46-47
18 Patient receives encouragement to participate in or to plan for the group's daily activities. ★D	18								48-49
19 The member of the group is provided with the opportunity to assume responsibility according to his capability. ★D	19								50-51
20 Staff proposals for patient activities appropriately reflect interest and needs of the group members. ★D	20								52-53
21 Patient is helped to vent his emotions in socially acceptable way within the group. ★D	21								54-55
22 Praise and recognition are given for achievement according to individual needs and with respect for others in the group. ★D	22								56-57
23 The rights and integrity of the group member are protected within the group structure. ★D	23								58-59
AREA II MEAN									60-61-62

PHYSICAL
Actions directed toward meeting physical needs of patients.

	Item number	Best care	Between	Average care	Between	Poorest care	Not applicable	Not observed	Mean score
24 Nursing procedures are adapted to meet needs of individual patient for treatment. ★D	24								63-64
25 Patient's daily hygiene needs for cleanliness and acceptable appearance are met. ★D	25								65-66
26 Nursing procedures are utilized as media for communication and interaction with patient. ★D	26								67-68
27 Physical symptoms and physical changes are identified and appropriate action taken. ★D	27								69-70
28 Physical distress evidenced by the patient is responded to quickly and appropriately. ★D	28								71-72
29 Patient is encouraged to observe appropriate rest & exercise. ★D/*I	29								73-74
30 Patient is encouraged to take adequate diet. ★D/*I	30								75-76
31 Action is taken to meet the patient's needs for adequate hydration and elimination. ★D/*I	31								77-78
32 Behavioural and physiologic changes due to medications are observed and appropriate action taken. ★D/*I	32								79-80
33 Expectations of patient's behaviour are adjusted and acted upon according to the effect the medication has on the patient. ★D/*I	33								11-12
34 Medical asepsis is carried out in relation to patient's personal hygiene and immediate environment. ★D	34								13-14
35 Medical and surgical asepsis is carried out during treatments and special procedures. ★D/*I	35								15-16
36 Environment is maintained that gives the patient a feeling of being safe and secure. ★D	36								17-18

Item number	Best care	Between	Average care	Between	Poorest care	Not applicable	Not observed	Mean score

37 Safety measures are carried out to prevent patient from harming himself or others. ★D

| 37 | | | | | | | | 19-20 |

38 Established techniques for safe administration of medications and parenteral fluids are carried out. ★D

| 38 | | | | | | | | 21-22 |

| AREA III MEAN | | | | | | | | 23-24-25 |

GENERAL
Actions that may be directed toward meeting either psychosocial or physical needs of the patient or both at the same time.

39 Patient receives instruction as necessary. ★D

| 39 | | | | | | | | 26-27 |

40 Patient and family are involved in planning for care and treatment. ★D/*I

| 40 | | | | | | | | 28-29 |

41 Patient's sensitivities and right to privacy are protected. ★D

| 41 | | | | | | | | 30-31 |

42 Patient is helped to accept dependence/independence as appropriate to his condition. ★D

| 42 | | | | | | | | 32-33 |

43 Resources within the milieu are utilised to provide the patient with opportunities for problem solving. ★D

| 43 | | | | | | | | 34-35 |

44 Patient is given freedom of choice in activities of daily living whenever possible and within patient's ability to make the choice. ★D

| 44 | | | | | | | | 36-37 |

45 Patient is encouraged to take part in activities of daily living that will stimulate his potential for positive psychosocial growth and movement toward physical independence. ★D/*I

| 45 | | | | | | | | 38-39 |

46 Activities are adapted to physical and mental capabilities of patient. ★D/*I

| 46 | | | | | | | | 40-41 |

47 Nursing care is adapted to patient's level and pace of development. ★D

| 47 | | | | | | | | 42-43 |

Item number	Best care	Between	Average care	Between	Poorest care	Not applicable	Not observed	Mean score

48 Diversional and/or treatment activities are made available to the patient according to his capabilities and needs. ★D

| 48 | | | | | | | | 44-45 |

49 Patient with slow or unskilled performance is accepted and encouraged. ★D

| 49 | | | | | | | | 46-47 |

50 Nursing care goals are established and activities performed which recognise and support the therapist's plan of care. ★D/*I

| 50 | | | | | | | | 48-49 |

51 Interaction with the patient is within the framework of the therapeutic plan. ★D

| 51 | | | | | | | | 50-51 |

52 Close observation of the patient is carried out with minimal disturbance. ★D

| 52 | | | | | | | | 52-53 |

53 Response to the patient is appropriate in emergency situations. ★D

| 53 | | | | | | | | 54-55 |

| AREA II MEAN | | | | | | | | 56-57-58 |

COMMUNICATION
Communication on behalf of the patient.

54 Ideas, facts, feelings and concepts about the patient are communicated clearly in speech to medical and paramedical personnel. ★D

| 54 | | | | | | | | 59-60 |

55 Family is provided with the opportunity for reciprocal communication with the nursing staff. ★D/*I

| 55 | | | | | | | | 61-62 |

56 Ideas, facts and concepts about the patient are clearly communicated in charting. *I

| 56 | | | | | | | | 63-64 |

57 Well-developed nursing care plans are established and incorporated into nursing assignments. *I

| 57 | | | | | | | | 65-66 |

58 Pertinent incidents of the patient's behaviour during interaction with staff are accurately reported. ★D/*I

| 58 | | | | | | | | 67-68 |

Item number	Best care	Between	Average care	Between	Poorest care	Not applicable	Not observed	Mean score

59 Staff participate in conferences concerning patient care.

| 59 | | | | | | | | 69-70 |

60 Effective communication and good relationships with other disciplines within the hospital are established for the patient's benefit.

| 60 | | | | | | | | 71-72 |

61 Patient's needs are met through the use of referrals, both to departments in the hospital and to other community agencies. ★D/*I

| 61 | | | | | | | | 73-74 |

| AREA V MEAN | | | | | | | | 75-76-77 |

PROFESSIONAL IMPLICATIONS
Care given to patient reflects initiative and responsibility indicative of professional expectations.

62 Decisions that are made by staff reflect knowledge of facts & good judgement. ★D/*I

| 62 | | | | | | | | 78-79 |

63 Evidence (spoken, behavioural, recorded) is given by staff of insight into deeper problems and needs of the patient. ★D/*I

| 63 | | | | | | | | 11-12 |

64 Changes in care and care plans reflect continuous evaluation of results of nursing care. ★D/*I

| 64 | | | | | | | | 13-14 |

65 Staff are reliable: follow through with responsibilities for the patient's care. ★D/*I

| 65 | | | | | | | | 15-16 |

66 Assigned staff keep informed of the patient's condition & whereabouts. ★D

| 66 | | | | | | | | 17-18 |

67 Care given the patient reflects flexibility in rules and regulations as indicated by individual patient needs. ★D/*I

| 67 | | | | | | | | 19-20 |

68 Organisation and management of nursing activities reflect due consideration for patient needs. ★D/*I

| 68 | | | | | | | | 21-22 |

| AREA VI MEAN | | | | | | | | 23-24-25 |

FINAL QUALPACS SCORE   Area I ☐   Area IV ☐
Area II ☐   Area V ☐
Area III ☐   Area· VI ☐
TOTAL ☐

Sum of item means		
Number of items rated		
Mean of item means		26-27-28

PART IV   CHART REVIEW SCHEDULE
(Please check in box of choice; DO NOT obscure number in box)

Name of patient: _____

            (last)   (first)

I   APPLICATION AND EXECUTION OF LEGAL MEDICAL PRESCRIPTIONS

	YES	NO	UNCERTAIN	TOTALS
1 Medical diagnosis complete	7	0	3	
2 Prescriptions complete	7	0	3	
3 Prescriptions current	7	0	3	
4 Prescriptions promptly executed	7	0	3	
5 Evidence that nurse understood cause and effect	7	0	3	
6 Evidence that nurse took health history into account	7	0	3	
(42) TOTALS		0		

II   OBSERVATION OF SYMPTOMS AND REACTIONS

	YES	NO	UNCERTAIN	TOTALS
7 Related to course of above condition in general	7	0	3	
8 Related to course of above condition in patient	7	0	3	
9 Related to complications due to therapy (each medication and each procedure)	7	0	3	
10 Vital signs	7	0	3	
11 Patient to his condition	7	0	3	
12 Patient to his course of disease(s)	7	0	2	
(40) TOTALS		0		

III   SUPERVISION OF THE PATIENT

	YES	NO	UNCERTAIN	TOTALS
13 Evidence that initial nursing problems were identified	4	0	1	
14 Safety of patient	4	0	1	
15 Security of patient	4	0	1	
16 Adaptation (support of patient in reaction to condition and care)	4	0	1	
17 Continuing assessment of patient's condition and capacity	4	0	1	
18 Nursing plans changed in accordance with assessment	4	0	1	
19 Interaction with family and with others considered	4	0	1	
(28) TOTALS		0		

IV   SUPERVISION OF THOSE PARTICIPATING IN CARE

	YES	NO	UNCERTAIN	TOTALS
20 Care taught to patient, family, or others, nursing personnel	5	0	2	
21 Physical, emotional, mental capacity to learn considered	5	0	2	
22 Continuity of supervision to those taught	5	0	2	
23 Support of those giving care	5	0	2	
(20) TOTALS		0		

V   REPORTING AND RECORDING

	YES	NO	UNCERTAIN	TOTALS
24 Facts on which further care depended were recorded	4	0	1	
25 Essential facts reported to doctor	4	0	1	
26 Reporting of facts included evaluation thereof	4	0	1	
27 Patient or family alerted as to what to report to doctor	4	0	1	
28 Record permitted continuity of intramural & extramural care	4	0	1	
(20) TOTALS		0		

VI APPLICATION AND EXECUTION OF NURSING PROCEDURES AND TECHNIQUES

	YES	NO	UNCERTAIN	TOTALS	DOES NOT APPLY
29 Administration and/or supervision of medications	2	0	0.5		2
30 Personal care (bathing, oral hygiene, skin, nail care, shampoo)	2	0	0.5		2
31 Nutrition (including special diets)	2	0	0.5		2
32 Fluid balance plus electrolytes	2	0	0.5		2
33 Elimination	2	0	0.5		2
34 Rest and sleep	2	0	0.5		2
35 Physical activity	2	0	0.5		2
36 Irrigations (including enemas)	2	0	0.5		2
37 Dressings and bandages	2	0	0.5		2
38 Formal exercise program	2	0	0.5		2
39 Rehabilitation (other than formal exercise)	2	0	0.5		2
40 Prevention of complications & infections	2	0	0.5		2
41 Recreation, diversion	2	0	0.5		2
42 Clinical procedures - urinalysis, B/P	2	0	0.5		2
43 Special treatments (eg care of tracheotomy, use of oxygen, colostomy or catheter care etc.)	2	0	0.5		2
44 Procedures and techniques taught to patient	2	0	0.5		2
(32) TOTALS		0			

VII PROMOTION OF PHYSICAL AND EMOTIONAL HEALTH BY DIRECTION AND TEACHING

	YES	NO	UNCERTAIN	TOTALS	DOES NOT APPLY
45 Plans for medical emergency evident	3	0	1		3
46 Emotional support to patient	3	0	1		3
47 Emotional support to family	3	0	1		3
48 Teaching promotion and maintenance of health	3	0	1		3
49 Evaluation of need for additional resources (e.g. spiritual, social service, home help service, phsio or occ. therapy)	3	0	1		3
50 Action taken in regard to needs identified (18) TOTALS	3	0	1		3

TOTAL SCORE

FINAL SCORE

AUDIT RESULTS
(All entries to be completed by a nursing audit committee member)

Record reflects service as:

Excellent (161–200)   Good (121–160)   Incomplete (81–120)   Poor (41–80)   Unsafe (0–40)
☐ (   )   ☐ (   )   ☐ (   )   ☐ (   )   ☐ (   )

Record did not permit appraisal ☐   Why?

Remarks (including criticisms/questions pertinent to policy procedures, practices as shown in Parts I and II):

_____   _____

Signature of Nursing Audit Committee member   Date
who reviewed the record

CUMULATIVE AUDIT REPORT

Number of records reviewed   ☐

Overall evaluation by number of cases   ☐   ☐   ☐   ☐   ☐

                              Excellent   Good   Incomplete   Poor   Unsafe

Evaluation by nursing function and number of cases

	Excellent	Good	Incomplete	Poor	Unsafe	TOTAL
(i) Application and execution of physician's legal orders						
(ii) Observation of symptoms and reactions						
(iii) Supervision of patient						
(iv) Supervision of those participating in care (except physician)						
(v) Reporting and recording						
(vi) Application and execution of nursing procedures and techniques						
(vii) Promotion of physical and emotional health by direction and teaching						

DIRECTIONS:

1   Overall results are summarised from Part III of completed audit schedules.

2   Results by function are summarised from Part II of completed audit schedules. For Functions I–V inclusive, use the final score attained; for Function VI and VII, use the final score attained PLUS the respective 'Does Not Apply' total. Relate the resulting to the judgment and resulting scores to the judgment and the scoring range below.

Function	Excellent	Good	Incomplete	Poor	Unsafe
I	36 – 42	27 – 35	18 – 26	9 – 17	0 – 8
II	32 – 40	24 – 31	16 – 23	8 – 15	0 – 7
III	23 – 28	16 – 22	10 – 15	5 – 9	0 – 4
IV	17 – 20	12 – 16	8 – 11	4 – 7	0 – 3
V	17 – 20	12 – 16	8 – 11	4 – 7	0 – 3
VII	16 – 18	12 – 15	8 – 11	4 – 7	0 – 3

PART V   PATIENT SERVICE CHECK LIST

Ask the patient whether the following statements are true/not true/not applicable.

		True	Not true	Not applicable	
1	The radio or TV was noisy	0	1	X	
2	My bed bath was not given to me when I wanted it	0	1	X	
3	The nurse was usually in a hurry	0	1	X	
4	Couldn't get anything from nurse for pain	0	1	X	
5	The nurse was prompt in answering my call	1	0	X	
6	Food trays were removed as soon as I was finished	1	0	X	
7	Thermometer left in too long	0	1	X	
8	Didn't see nurse often enough	0	1	X	
9	My bedpan or commode was removed promptly	1	0	X	
10	My food was served at the right temperature	1	0	X	
11	Nurse or assistants left me with clean towels	1	0	X	
12	My meals were served as I had ordered	1	0	X	
13	Drinking water was changed regularly	1	0	X	
14	Other patients made disturbing noises	0	1	X	
15	Nurse left before I could ask her question	0	1	X	
16	Had to wait too long for a bedpan	0	1	X	
17	The nurses offered to stay with me when I was first allowed up	1	0	X	
18	The nurses fed me when I needed help	1	0	X	
19	My room was comfortable to sleep in	1	0	X	
20	I was not propped up, making it hard to enjoy my meal	0	1	X	
21	The nurses never told me how they were going to care for me	1	0	X	
22	The nurses let me do things at my own speed	0	1	X	
23	The nurses offered to bathe me when I needed help	0	1	X	
24	Light was too bright when I tried to sleep	0	1	X	
25	The hallways near my room were fairly quiet	1	0	X	
26	Nurses seemed very interested in me	1	0	X	
27	Bathroom was not clean	0	1	X	
28	My bath, meal or rest period was interrupted by treatment	0	1	X	
29	If I felt bad, I was not asked to do anything I didn't want to	1	0	X	
30	I was awakened to have my temperature taken	0	1	X	
31	Was not served drinks after I requested them	0	1	X	
32	In general, my room was neat and tidy	1	0	X	
33	The nurses wouldn't tell me what was wrong with me	0	1	X	
34	My food was cold when served	0	1	X	
35	The nurses were very nice to me	1	0	X	
36	The nurses were with me fairly often	1	0	X	
37	Bed was not changed often enough	0	1	X	
38	The patients near me were fairly quiet	1	0	X	
39	Nurse did not wash and rub my back well	0	1	X	

	True	Not true	Not applicable	
40 The nurse was not prompt in answering my call	1	0	X	
41 Air in my room was always fresh	1	0	X	
42 I didn't get medicine when I requested it	0	1	X	
43 The nurses take their time with me	1	0	X	
44 My bandage or dressing was too tight	0	1	X	
45 Bedpan was brought to me promptly	1	0	X	
46 I was given a wheelchair when I asked for one	1	0	X	

Total Score

Score items = 46 – not applicable ratings

Total score ÷ scored items

Total patient service score (= six final scores ÷ 6)

PART VI   QUALITY ASSESSMENT SUMMARY

FINAL QUALITY ASSESSMENT SCORE

1   Structure

General comments:

Structural review score   ☐

2   Process

General comments:

Qualpacs score   ☐

Audit score   ☐

3   Outcome

General comments:

Patient Service Checklist score   ☐

Index